The 7-Da  Reflux Diet

Cure Acid Reflux, GERD and Heartburn NOW with the Easy to Follow Lifestyle, Diet and 45 Mouth-Watering Recipes

Robert M. Fleischer

NaturalWay Publishing

Atlanta, Georgia USA

ISBN 978-1-484994-29-0

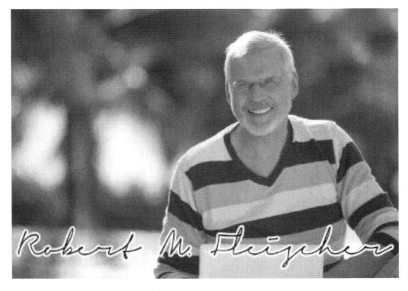

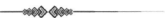

Praises from Readers

"I've suffered from GERD for years without knowing. This book has opened my eyes to the realities of the disease and helped my health in more than one ways."

★★★★☆ Laura Stokes (Ocala, FL)

"I'm grateful for books like this one that help us get to know our bodies better and help us find our way out of dire circumstances."

★★★★★ Katherine C. Reilly (Panama City, FL)

"GERD sounds like a joke, but it's not. It's painful and it can wear you down. Thanks to this book relief is now just a few mouse clicks away."

★★★★☆ Yolanda Barker (Deer River, NY)

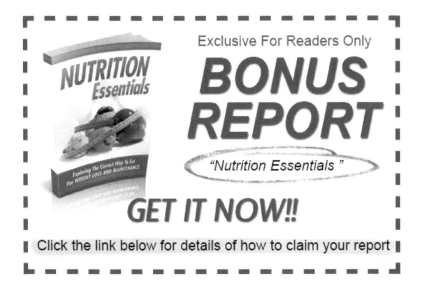
Exclusive Bonus Download: Nutrition Essentials

Get All The Support And Guidance You Need To Be A Success At Understanding Nutrition!

Is the fact that you would like to get a grip on how to understand how to eat right for a healthy weight but just don't know how making your life difficult... maybe even miserable?

First, you are NOT alone! It may seem like it sometimes, but not knowing how to get started with nutrition for a healthy weight is far more common than you'd think.

Your lack of knowledge in this area may not be your fault, but that doesn't mean that you shouldn't -- or can't -- do anything to find out everything you need to know to finally be a success with understanding nutrition to have better health!

So today -- in the next FEW MINUTES, in fact -- we're going to help you GET ON TRACK, and learn how you can

4

quickly and easily get your nutrition issues under control... for GOOD!

With this product, and it's great information on nutrition will walk you, step by step, through the exact process we developed to help people get all the info they need to be a success.

In This Book, You Will Learn:

- The Food Pyramid
- Correct Proteins For Weight Loss
- Correct Carbs For Weight Loss
- Correct Fats For Weight Loss
- What About Organic And Raw Foods
- And so much more!

<u>Download this guide and start living healthily **NOW**</u>

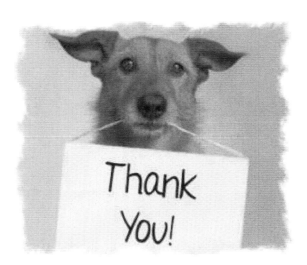

Thank you for downloading my book. Please REVIEW this book on Amazon. I need your feedback to make the next version better. Thank you so much!

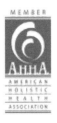

Author Foreword

The gastroesophageal reflux disease or GERD is an illness that can affect generations of people that belong to the same family, a lot of whom may lead for long a life in pain, as its symptoms may remind them of something else; a less serious disease.

My book comes as a practical guide to all those people who suffer from GERD. It is a common illness and it usually occurs when the lower esophageal sphincter isn't functioning correctly. That can make the patient feel extreme pain in the chest in some cases, while in others it develops different, but no less painful symptoms.

So, the first question that comes to mind is: "What can someone do to get better?" You can find the answer to that question and much more in the pages of this book, as within them I present various treatments, from detoxification to dietary changes and acupuncture. At the same time I propose a specific schedule you can follow, which can help improve your bodily functions and state of mind.

GERD, despite its weird acronym, is not one of those diseases that one should take lightly. So, read, learn, follow the instructions, and go on to lead a long and healthy life.

Table of Contents

Disclaimer

While all attempts have been made to provide effective, verifiable information in this Book, neither the Author nor Publisher assumes any responsibility for errors, inaccuracies, or omissions. Any slights of people or organizations are unintentional.

This Book is not a source of medical information, and it should not be regarded as such. This publication is designed to provide accurate and authoritative information in regard to the subject matter covered. It is sold with the understanding that the publisher is not engaged in rendering a medical service. As with any medical advice, the reader is strongly encouraged to seek professional medical advice before taking action.

1. The Basics

1.1. What is GERD?

The Center for Women's Health tells the story of Gloria, a 53-year-old woman who was experiencing a burning in her chest. She felt like she always had a lump in her throat, and an acidic taste in the back of her mouth. Sound unpleasant? Gloria had been dealing with this not for a few days or weeks, but for several years. After a while, she started to worry that these were symptoms of a serious problem, like heart disease, so she saw her doctor. Fortunately, her doctor told her that her symptoms were not indicative of heart disease, but that she was most likely experiencing GERD.

When you hear someone talk about heartburn, they often talk about acid reflux or 'GERD', which is an awfully complicated-sounding acronym. So what, exactly, does GERD stand for? It stands for gastroesophageal reflux disease (you can see why someone would want to turn this into an acronym; it's a mouthful). Now, what does *that* mean? Let's break it down, and take it one word at a time. First 'gastroesophageal'. 'Gastro', as you may have guessed, means 'having to do with the stomach', and 'esophageal', obviously, relates to the esophagus, the tube that connects your mouth to your stomach (this is the tube through which food passes—and, as we shall see, through which gastric acid might also pass). 'Reflux' means 'a passing back', and refers to the movement of gastric acid back through the esophagus. 'Disease', the final word in the acronym, is pretty self-explanatory.

So there you have it—GERD is a disorder in which gastric acid passes from the stomach into the esophagus, causing discomfort.

Why does gastric acid in the esophagus cause such pain? Because it's not meant to be there. The stomach has a lining that can resist the strong acids that are used for digestion, but the esophagus isn't designed for that, and having the acid in the esophagus is painful.

Okay, so we've defined gastroesophageal reflux disease. Now, what are acid reflux and heartburn? Acid reflux is just another term for GERD—acid going where it shouldn't. Heartburn, however, is a symptom of the disease, and describes the pain you may feel after eating, caused by the gastric acid in the esophagus. It seems obvious where the name comes from—if you've ever experienced heartburn, you know that it's best described as a burning sensation in your chest, somewhere around where your heart is. Even though it has nothing to do with your heart, it's a fitting name for this type of pain.

1.2. What causes GERD?

Generally, the body is very good at keeping gastric acid in the stomach where it belongs—so why do some people experience heartburn? While the ultimate cause may vary between different people, one thing is certain: the lower esophageal sphincter, which usually keeps the esophagus closed to stomach acids, isn't functioning correctly. You can think of the lower esophageal sphincter as a valve that allows food to pass from the esophagus to the stomach while keeping the contents of the stomach from backing up into the esophagus. If this valve isn't working correctly, bad things happen. Basically, the cause of the problem is that the sphincter isn't closed tight enough (or, in more technical terms, doesn't have enough muscular tone), and the valve becomes a two-way passage instead of a unidirectional one.

1.3. Risk factors for reflux disease

'But *why*,' you might be asking, 'does the sphincter not work correctly?' This is a valid question, but a much more difficult one to answer. Research shows that genetics might be to blame; a 2007 study in Northern Ireland showed that adolescents were significantly more likely to experience heartburn if their parents also experienced it, and this correlation was even stronger when both parents had problems with acid reflux. So if you're struggling with acid reflux, you might have your parents to blame. There are other risk factors, too. The Mayo Clinic lists the following, among others:

- Obesity
- Smoking
- Pregnancy
- Asthma
- Diabetes

Let's take these one at a time, as the connection between some of these conditions and acid reflux might not be very intuitive. First, obesity. Researchers aren't totally sure why obesity has such a marked connection to GERD, but they have a few theories. Extra pressure on the stomach from excess body fat might push gastric acid back into the esophagus, too many fatty foods might alter the acid in the stomach or relax the lower esophageal sphincter, and people whose body mass index (BMI) is in the obese category are more likely to develop hernias, which can also increase the risk of reflux. Smoking reduces the strength and muscle tone of the lower esophageal sphincter, making it more likely that it will not close correctly (coincidentally, alcohol has a similar effect). Pregnancy, like obesity, has a less well-understood, though significant, connection to GERD. A developing baby might put extra pressure on the stomach, pushing gastric acid through the esophageal valve, and hormonal changes that affect muscle tone in the uterus might also affect the sphincter, not allowing it to maintain proper closure. These hormonal changes may also slow the digestion in your stomach. Although the connection between asthma and acid reflux isn't clear, it does appear to be a complicated one—it's not certain if one causes the other, or if they exacerbate each other, or if acid reflux simply interferes with the pharmaceutical treatments for asthma. What *is* clear, however, is that having asthma means you are more likely to experience acid reflux. The relationship between diabetes and GERD isn't well understood either, but it appears that having Type 2 diabetes does increase your risk for acid reflux, even apart from being overweight (which is a risk factor for Type 2 diabetes).

All of these things, and more, may contribute to an increased risk of gastroesophageal reflux disease. Another significant one is medications; there are certain types of medications—some pretty common ones among them—that can increase the severity of acid reflux and possibly cause it in the first place. Several heart medications, including calcium channel blockers (which include Norvasc and Plendil) and nitrates (like Dilatrate, Isordil, and Nitrolingual), have been indicated in increasing the risk of acid reflux. Other drugs that might cause or worsen GERD include theophylline (for asthma), narcotics (usually painkillers, like codeine, Vicodin, and Lortab), sedatives (including Valium and other sleeping pills), and supplementary progesterone (which may be prescribed to women who are pregnant or trying to get pregnant). As you can see, the list of medications that could complicate matters is quite long, so if you're taking any medications, make sure to discuss the risk of possible complications with your doctor.

If you're suffering from heartburn, you know that certain foods seem to bring it on. Because of this, there are a lot of foods that should be avoided if you experience acid reflux. WebMD lists the top 10 heartburn foods as follows:

- Tangy citrus fruits
- Tomatoes
- Garlic and onion
- Spicy foods
- Peppermint
- Cheese, nuts, avocados, and meat
- Alcohol
- Caffeine
- Chocolate
- Carbonated beverages

As you can see, these are foods that are quite common in the Western diet. A lot of these foods are very acidic, like the citrus fruits and tomatoes, but some of the others might surprise you. For example, #6 doesn't contain spicy or acidic foods, but foods that are high in fat, which slow emptying of the stomach, and can result in increased pressure on the lower esophageal sphincter. The spicy foods on the list seem pretty self-explanatory; if your mouth feels like it's burning when you put a food into it, don't put that food into your stomach if you're at risk for GERD! Several of the other foods, including alcohol and peppermint, are likely to relax the esophageal valve and allow gastric acid into your esophagus.

Making dietary changes isn't always easy, but if you're suffering from painful heartburn, making the effort to cut out foods that make it worse will be worth it. Adopting a diet that is focused on easing your troubles with acid reflux (such as the one that is detailed in chapter 3) could help treat this very painful condition.

1.4 Candida

The digestive system is home to a great many types of bacteria, most of which are beneficial and contribute to the proper functioning of your body, like peptostrococcus, Clostridium, and E. coli. Among these beneficial bacteria is Candida albicans. However, Candida overgrowth has been implicated in many gastrointestinal problems, including abdominal pain, cramping, irritable bowel syndrome (IBS), and indigestion, as well as more serious issues like GERD, urinary tract infections, and even food allergies. While there are different theories as to why Candida is related to heartburn, it seems pretty clear that there's some relation, and that treating significant Candida overgrowth can improve your health and prevent potentially serious complications from the overgrowth spreading to the rest of your body.

Why does Candida overgrowth occur? There are many possible reasons. Taking a course of antibiotics, for example, can disrupt the natural balance of bacteria in your body and create an environment that is amenable to Candida albicans. Disordered gastric acid production, as well as being caused *by* Candida overgrowth, can also *cause* Candida overgrowth, prolonging the cycle. More commonly, however, a Candida overgrowth is caused by a slight disruption in the balance of the body in combination with a diet high in foods that feed the bacteria. What feeds Candida? Unfortunately, many of the common foods in the Western diet. Processed meats, milk and cheese, starchy vegetables, many caffeinated beverages, almost anything that contains gluten, nearly any kind of sugar that you can think of, and even artificial sweeteners like aspartame, acesulfame, and sucralose (so replacing Coke with Diet Coke won't help you much when it comes to Candida).

If Candida is one of the contributing factors to your GERD, you're going to have to adopt a detoxifying diet to help your digestive system reset and cleanse itself to get Candida under control. A diet like this will starve Candida of its primary sources of food, allowing your body to combat the overgrowth and reduce its population to a proper level. In addition to dietary changes, there are anti-Candida supplements that you can take to specifically target the overgrowth. For more information on these strategies, see chapter 3, section 4.

1.5 Signs and symptoms

Although the symptoms of gastroesophageal reflux disease vary from person to person, there are a few tell-tale signs, the first among them being heartburn. If you get a painful burning sensation in the center of your chest, behind your breastbone, you're likely experiencing heartburn that could be caused by acid reflux. You may also get a sour or bitter taste in your throat that comes from acid being regurgitated into your esophagus. In an attempt to get your acid reflux under control, your body may start producing an overabundance of saliva, which you may notice. All of the aforementioned symptoms are likely to occur after eating. These symptoms are quite common, and are usually enough to indicate that you're experiencing at least mild GERD.

More severe symptoms are less common, though certainly not unheard of. Inflammation and irritation of the throat is one—understandably, the linings of your organs are irritated by the caustic acid from your stomach, and can cause a sore throat. If this inflammation is bad and the regurgitation is serious, you can experience vomiting or nausea as well. It's possible for gastric acid to irritate the nerves running throughout your body, leading to inflammation in the lungs, coughing, and possible exacerbation of asthma. Although it's extremely unlikely, you may also experience chest or neck pain, in which case you should immediately seek advice from your doctor.

It should be noted that, although most sufferers of GERD are adults, it sometimes occurs in children and infants as well, who show some different symptoms. According to WebMD, infants and children may exhibit frequent or recurring vomiting or cough, refuse to eat, cry while eating or feeding, or express abdominal pain (though obviously pre-verbal infants have difficulty this). Reflux is common in infants, and they usually outgrow it in their first year of age, though it's still worth bringing it up with your pediatrician if you think your child is experiencing acid reflux.

Of course, some people experience uncommon symptoms. For example, one woman, after taking an intense course of antibiotics, experienced inflammation in her upper palate (the hard part at the top of the back of your mouth), swollen lymph nodes, a lump in her throat, and chronic fatigue. She was so tired that she slept twelve hours a day! When she saw her doctor, he told her that she likely had an acid reflux disorder. Not all of this woman's symptoms were typical of GERD, but seeing a doctor helped her discover that she was suffering from acid reflux.

1.6. Diagnosing GERD

There are quite a few different ways to conclusively diagnose GERD, but they're often not needed, as the combination of heartburn after eating and acid regurgitation (which is what causes the sour or bitter taste in your throat) are quite indicative of the disorder. However, it's always good to conduct tests to ensure an accurate diagnosis. Although this is a pretty comprehensive list of diagnostic procedures, it's always possible that your doctor will have another one in mind, or a new one will be developed. For this overview, we'll start with the least invasive procedure and go from there.

1. Throat and larynx examination.

Because acid reflux causes inflammation of the throat and larynx (this is what can cause a cough or hoarseness), this is a good place to start. An ear, nose, and throat (ENT) specialist will look at your throat to see if you show any of the signs of inflammation. Whether they see anything or not, they may progress to a more accurate test after this.

2. Proton pump inhibitor test.

Another minimally invasive procedure, this simply involves the swallowing of a medication that suppresses the acid in your stomach. If your symptoms go away, and then come back when you stop the medication, it's a good sign that you're suffering from acid reflux.

3. Barium swallow radiograph test.

This sounds a lot worse than it is. All you have to do is drink a barium solution (which might not be terribly pleasant, but it's not too bad), and then doctors will monitor its movement through your body with an x-ray machine. The barium makes it clear on the x-rays if there are abnormalities with how food and other substances travel through your body.

4. Gastric emptying study.

Similar to the barium test, this involves a slightly radioactive substance. This time, however, you eat a meal that includes the substance, and doctors will monitor how long it takes for food to exit your stomach. As was mentioned above, if food stays in your stomach too long, it can contribute to acid reflux, so this is a good way to gain some insight into how long it takes.

5. pH monitoring.

A small tube is inserted into the esophagus, and left there for one or two days. This sounds awfully uncomfortable but, other than a slight gagging sensation during the insertion, you should be relatively comfortable. While the tube is in place, you will wear a monitor on the outside of your body that records the amount of acid that enters your esophagus. Because it directly measures the acid levels in your esophagus, this is considered by some to be the gold-standard test for GERD.

6. Esophageal manometry.

This is similar to the pH monitoring, but this time, a catheter is swallowed for an hour or so, and it monitors the muscle tone of your esophagus, and can reveal whether or not your lower esophageal sphincter is experiencing problems.

7. Upper endoscopy exam.

Because this exam involves the use of an endoscope—a small tube with a tiny camera on the end—it can provide the doctors with a first-hand look at what's going on in your esophagus. Although the procedure is quite invasive, you'll be anesthetized or sedated enough so that you're very relaxed and comfortable. If the results of this indicate it, a full endoscopy exam may take place, which includes your stomach and small intestine—this can reveal many different problems that are related to acid reflux that are difficult to diagnose through other methods.

As you can see, there are many ways of diagnosing gastroesophageal reflux disease, all of which have their merits. Which test your doctor chooses depends on the severity of your symptoms as well as which tests are easily available.

1.7 Complications of reflux disease

So we've established that acid reflux is a painful disorder. But is there more to it? Are there more serious side effects of GERD than discomfort, or is it simply an irritation? Turns out that acid in the esophagus can cause more than just heartburn.

The presence of gastric acid in the esophagus causes inflammation (which you've experienced elsewhere before—if you've had an infected cut, and it's turned red, and gotten warm, and painful to the touch, that was inflammation at work), which, by itself, isn't a big deal. It's painful, and can be awfully annoying, as you use your esophagus all the time, but the inflammation itself isn't dangerous.

If left untreated, however, GERD can allow too much corrosive gastric acid into the esophagus, which can eat away at the esophageal lining and cause ulcers, or holes in the esophagus. As if this wasn't bad enough, if the ulcers are very severe, they can cause internal bleeding that requires serious medical intervention, as this is very dangerous, even life-threatening, in its most severe form. Most people think of ulcers as just being painful and annoying—kind of like acid reflux—but it's important to know that they can also have serious effects.

The long-term effects of inflammation and ulcers can also result in scarring of the esophagus, which can eventually lead to a narrowing of the esophagus, a condition called stricture. This narrowing can interfere with the passage of food and liquids through the esophagus, a problem that can be solved surgically or through a process called dilation, in which the esophagus is stretched. Although strictures aren't in themselves dangerous, the treatments for them are significant and unpleasant, and if you can avoid esophageal scarring, you should make an effort to.

One of the most serious complications of reflux disease is called Barrett's esophagus; this is a very complicated sequence of events that usually starts with chronic heartburn (though, in rare cases, people who experience no heartburn can develop it) and ends with abnormal cells lining the esophagus. The exact mechanism of this change is quite complicated, but the end result is that the cells that line the esophagus harden, making it very difficult for food to pass into the stomach. What's more, people who suffer from Barrett's esophagus are significantly more likely to develop esophageal cancer. Because of the danger of Barrett's esophagus, it's important to have endoscopic screenings if you suffer from chronic heartburn, so that any potentially serious problems can be detected early and treated or prevented.

There are additional complications outside of the esophagus. According to WebMD, uncontrolled chronic heartburn may also contribute to chronic lung problems, including bronchitis, emphysema, and coughing (likely due to the spreading of inflammation from the esophagus to the lungs). In addition to these debilitating effects, heartburn may also cause voice and throat problems, as well as dental erosion from harsh acids entering the mouth.

To sum it up, a lot of bad things can happen if you experience chronic gastroesophageal reflux disease and don't get it under control. Fortunately for anyone who's suffering from this painful condition, there are many treatments available, each of which has its own strengths and weaknesses.

1.8 Conventional treatment

When it comes to treating GERD there are two main types of treatment: conventional and alternative. Conventional treatments include some of the things discussed in the preceding sections, like medications and surgery. Alternative treatments involve non-traditional means that are based on a holistic view of the body, which means that practitioners of alternative medicine believe that disorders stem from certain weaknesses in the body's natural immune system. These weaknesses are then treated by a variety of methods (more on that in chapter 3). Practitioners of alternative medicine (also called 'natural' or 'holistic' medicine) believe that conventional methods do not take the body into account as a whole and complete system, but only address specific issues in specific organs, regardless of where the problem begins.

Some conventional treatments are ones you've probably heard of. Antacids, for example, are a common way to try to treat heartburn. Over-the-counter antacids, like Alka-Seltzer, milk of magnesia, Pepto-Bismol, and Mylanta, reduce the acidity of the gastric acids so that they don't cause damage or inflammation when they enter the esophagus. As you might imagine, this does very little to address the causes of heartburn, and simply masks the primary symptom. They can, however, be useful in reducing the pain caused by ulcers, which is exacerbated by stomach acids.

Histamine antagonists, or H2 blockers, such as Zantac, Tagamet, and Pepcid, suppress acid production in the stomach. This is a different mechanism of action than antacids, but it has a similar effect. They are sometimes taken in conjunction with antacids to provide additional protection. There is one medication, Pepcid Complete, which contains both an H2 blocker and an antacid. Proton pump inhibitors, another class of drugs, also work to block acid production in the stomach. Prevacid, Prilosec, and Nexium are examples of this type of drug.

All of the drugs listed above are used to treat mild-to-moderate acid reflux, but are also available in prescription strengths to treat more severe symptoms (though because they focus on treating the symptoms of GERD, and not the cause, they are generally recommended for non-chronic sufferers of acid reflux). Both the over-the-counter and prescription-strength versions of these drugs should only be taken under the direction of a doctor, as overuse of them can cause various adverse side effects.

A different class of drugs, prokinetics, is often combined with the medications listed above, but has a very different way of treating acid reflux—it gets closer to the source of the problem, and helps increase the muscle tone that's lacking in the lower esophageal sphincter, as well as speeding the emptying of the stomach. While this may sound like a good way to treat GERD, these medications often have very serious side effects that could outweigh their usefulness in treating acid reflux.

In very serious cases, doctors might advocate a more intense form of conventional medicine—surgery. This is generally only recommended in extreme cases that are not ameliorated by medications and pose a serious risk to the patient's health (as is sometimes the case when inflammation spreads to the lungs). There are different types of surgery, but most of them aim to accomplish the same thing: reinforcing of the lower valve of the esophagus using the upper folds of the stomach. Though this surgery can be quite successful, it is also risky, as it may cause side effects that cannot be relieved, even with a second surgery.

There are many natural, holistic remedies for GERD, many of which will be discussed below. The next chapter will focus on a few simple strategies that you can make to quickly help improve heartburn, acid reflux, and other symptoms you may be having. Chapter 3 will focus on providing you with an outline of a complete holistic treatment plan for getting your body back in balance to treat GERD. Chapter 4 discusses some additional alternative treatments you should consider. Finally, Chapter 5 includes a selection of recipes for inclusion in your anti-GERD diet.

2. Emergency 7-Day Treatment Strategies

Before laying out the full plan for managing your gastroesophageal reflux disease, I'll provide you with a short plan that will help you cure (or at least very significantly reduce) your symptoms. Heartburn is a painful and irritating thing, and when you're suffering from it, you want to act fast—so here are some fast tips for getting rid of your symptoms quickly. Of course, this is only a temporary treatment. While all of these points will hold true during your long-term management of acid reflux, there's a lot more to it, and you should continue with the holistic treatment plan outlined in chapter 3. However, this is a good place to start, and should have you feeling better within a week. Also, it's important to note that while this is called an 'emergency treatment' plan, it's not for any sort of medical emergency. If you're feeling neck or chest pain due to your heartburn, or you have serious issues with your GERD, contact an emergency medical provider or call 911 immediately.

2.1. Detoxify Your Diet

Although there are many different reasons for heartburn, food is at the core of a lot of them. Obviously, a condition that is centered in your stomach and esophagus is going to be highly affected by food, and the first step to quick relief of heartburn is by getting your diet under control. Remember that the dietary strategies presented here are for short-term relief of acid reflux symptoms—this isn't a diet that you'll have to stick to for a long period of time. It's basically a more intense version of the dietary changes presented in chapter 3, which is part of a long-term, holistic plan to get your body back in balance. The diet suggested here should only be undertaken for a week before you start slowly reintroducing other foods back into your diet. It is, essentially, a detoxifying diet that will help your reset your digestive system.

On to the strategies. Below are five guidelines to follow for the week of your detoxification. The strategies discussed below will allow your body to cleanse itself of the by-products of the harmful foods you've been consuming throughout most of your life. Because of this, you may experience some discomfort—your stomach may be a little upset (bloating, gas, etc.), and your digestive system may not seem to be working correctly (you may have altered bowel movements), but stick with it and everything will get back to normal. Better than normal, in fact, because you won't be feeling heartburn after every meal.

Of course, you should consult a doctor before adopting any dietary changes.

1. Cut out animal products.

This means no meat, no fish, no cheese, and no dairy products—not even lean ones. No poultry or even low-fat dairy. All of this has to go to ensure that your digestive system is able to cleanse itself properly. This is going to be challenging for most people, but don't worry; you'll be able to consume moderate amounts of most of these foods once you've completed the 7-day emergency plan. One way that you can get some protein (as well as many other beneficial nutrients) during this phase is by adding nuts, including almonds and Brazil nuts, to your diet (sunflower and pumpkin seeds are good, too).

2. Cut out trigger foods.

In addition to animal products, there are many foods that generally exacerbate heartburn. Obviously, everyone has their own trigger foods, but there are quite a few that seem to be generally irritating to the stomach and esophagus. These include spicy foods, highly processed foods, white sugar, and products that contain caffeine, chocolate, tobacco, or alcohol. Again, you may be able to add some of these back into your diet later, but for now, you'll be much better off just completely cutting them out.

3. Increase fruits and vegetables.

Most people don't get nearly enough fruits or vegetables in their daily diet. If you're going to treat heartburn, you have to change this and start getting enough produce. Any produce is good, but a few types are best: things like apples, grapes, spinach, carrots, and other non-citrus, non-starchy fruits and vegetables. And you can never go wrong with eating green, leafy vegetables. Part of what you're trying to accomplish here is to get your gastric acids back in balance, so eating acidic foods isn't going to help.

4. Reduce gluten-based grains.

Wheat, barley, rye, and other similar grains contain gluten, which can cause problems for your digestive system. Adopting a gluten-free diet for a few days will help your body return to its proper state. Even after the emergency treatment plan is over, you should consider adopting a gluten-free diet. Many people have given testimonies about how they feel better—physically, mentally, and emotionally— after eliminating gluten.

5. Add pseudograins.

The seeds of pseudograins, like quinoa, amaranth, buckwheat, and chia, are better for you than the traditional cereal grains. Because these plants are biologically different from cereal grains, your body processes them differently, and the resulting effects are much less unpleasant. Fortunately, it's easy to replace almost any grain with a pseudograin (if you're stuck for ideas on how to replace some things that seem like they just can't be made without wheat, like pizza crust, cookies, or pancakes, try looking up recipes for them online; many websites that feature Paleo diet recipes will provide suitable alternatives to traditional recipes for these foods).

6. Drink a lot of water.

In addition to keeping you hydrated, water helps flush toxins out of your body, which is crucial during this phase of the emergency treatment. It's a good practice, not just during the cleansing period, to drink a glass of water as soon as you wake up in the morning, and another before you go to bed. Keep a water bottle with you throughout the day, and sip on it regularly. Have a glass with each meal. The Mayo Clinic states that, on average, men need three liters (about 13 cups) of water a day, while women need around 2.2 liters (9 cups) each day. Everyone has their own requirements, and it depends a great deal on your body size, your level of activity, and other individual factors. Sticking to the Mayo recommendations is a great start, though.

To be blunt, undertaking a detoxifying diet is not easy. In fact, it might be quite unpleasant for a day or two. However, after you complete the first round of detoxification, you will start to feel a great deal better, and you may even decide to adopt several of these guidelines to your normal diet.

2.2 Supplement Your Diet

Candida albicans, as mentioned in section 4 of chapter 1, can contribute not only to your gastroesophageal reflux disease, but to many other painful and dangerous conditions as well. So making sure that the Candida in your body is not in a state of overgrowth is crucial in getting your heartburn under control, especially in the emergency treatment phase. If there's too much Candida in your system, making dietary changes is only going to solve half the problem—you have to eliminate the bacteria before you can get your system back into balance.

Before detailing the supplements that you can take to kill off Candida overgrowth, it's also important to note that you should attempt to clear your system of as many harmful parasites and bacteria as possible during this phase. There are billions of bacteria in your body, but there could also be more insidious parasites living in your digestive tract that you aren't aware of, and these can contribute to GERD, so it's crucial to take them all out in one fell swoop. To this end, you should take some of the following supplements during the first days of your emergency treatment, *before* starting your anti-Candida supplements. Of course, adding supplements to your daily routine is something that should be discussed with your doctor, especially if you're already taking other supplements or prescription medications.

The first anti-parasite supplement to add to your diet is garlic. You can get it in capsule or tablet form or, of course, in cloves. Unfortunately, garlic may exacerbate your heartburn, so be careful while taking it—you don't want to cause more damage than has already been done, even if garlic is one of the more effective anti-parasite remedies. Goldenseal, an herb, is a long-standing treatment for many types of infections, and can help clear your digestive system (and the rest of your body) of harmful parasites. Although the safety and effectiveness of black walnut and wormwood have not been evaluated in clinical trials, they are known in folk medicine to be effective against intestinal parasites, and can be found in several forms.

Once you've started to clear parasites from your body, you can focus on Candida. While some of the above remedies might help clear Candida, there are more focused supplements that you can take to specifically target the bacteria. There are many different supplements that you can take, but stick with one or two to avoid interactions and complications. If you started taking garlic or goldenseal to cleanse your body of parasites, you can continue taking it, as they can also help with the Candida. Other herbal supplements include echinacea, oregano (in enteric-coated capsules), peppermint (in enteric-coated capsules), and rosemary oil (again, in enteric-coated capsules). Non-herbal supplements include betaine hydrochloride and other digestive enzymes, as well as caprylic acid. All of these supplements should help get the bacteria in your digestive system back in balance, and help prevent Candida from causing more problems.

It's important to mention again that taking supplements is something that you should discuss with your doctor before beginning. It's also good to take general supplements throughout the course of your GERD treatment—things like multivitamins, B and C complexes, EFA, colostrum, and chlorella.

2.3. Replenish Beneficial Bacteria

One of the unfortunate side effects of cleansing your body of parasites and Candida is that you will also inadvertently remove many of the beneficial bacteria that routinely inhabit your digestive system. After completing the course of anti-parasite and anti-Candida supplements, it's important to provide your body with the proper substances to help these good bacteria re-colonize your stomach and small intestine. There are two ways of doing this, and by combining them, you can help ensure the success of this step.

First, add pre-biotic foods to your diet. You've probably heard about pro-biotics, but pre-biotics are a little less popular. While a pro-biotic contains bacteria that are beneficial to your digestive system, a pre-biotic contains nutrients that feed the bacteria that are already present in your system (this is important, because some studies have found that the bacteria in pro-biotics have difficulty surviving the trip to the stomach. While there are many different foods that contain pre-biotic nutrients, it's best to avoid the ones that might exacerbate your heartburn. Onions, garlic, leeks, and artichokes are good pre-biotic foods that shouldn't upset your stomach too much.

In addition to these pre-biotic foods, you should also take pro-biotic supplements to help replenish the beneficial bacteria in your body. While there are foods that have been supplemented with pro-biotic bacteria, a large number of them are in the dairy category, which is one that you should be cutting out during your 7-day treatment, so you should avoid those (if you find that you're able to add dairy back into your diet later, these are good options). You should stick to pro-biotic supplements that you can find at your local natural foods store, or ones that your doctor recommends to you.

2.4. Control Stress

Once you've detoxified your diet, gotten rid of excess Candida albicans, and encouraged the beneficial bacteria in your body to return to healthy levels, you're almost all the way through your 7-day cleanse and heartburn treatment. There's just one crucial step left, but it might be one of the most difficult: control your stress. While research is equivocal, there's definitely evidence that supports the idea that stress is a contributor to GERD. Even if stress isn't specifically contributing your symptoms, it's likely at the root of some other issues in your life, so it's a good idea to get it under control anyway. You may not know it, but experiencing chronic stress can take a huge toll on both your body and your mind, and to get them both functioning optimally, you need to manage it.

How do you manage stress? This is a huge question, and the answer varies from person to person. Stress is caused by situational and environmental factors, so there's no strategy that will work equally well for everyone. A good first step is to think about the stressors in your life—are you stressed by your job? Your health? Your crazy schedule? What's contributing to your stress level? Once you've identified the sources of your stress, you can begin to take action to reduce it.

However, since you can't completely address these issues over night, I will list a few strategies that will help you get your stress under control in the short term. First, meditate. It might sound crazy, and you might think that it's a waste of time, but if you commit to trying it for the 7 days of your treatment, you may find that it makes a world of difference. When you wake up in the morning, after having a glass of water, sit quietly for ten to fifteen minutes. Sit in a quiet room, close your eyes, and just concentrate on your breathing. Try to totally clear your mind of everything else—focus on the slow, gentle, in, out, in, out of your breath. Don't think about what's on your schedule for the day, or what your kids will eat for breakfast. Don't worry about work. Just think about breathing. After fifteen minutes of this, your mind will be clearer, more relaxed, and better prepared to start the day.

In addition to once-daily (or even better, twice-daily) meditation, you should also make a point to exercise at least a few times a week (the Centers for Disease Control recommends two-and-a-half hours of moderate-intensity exercise each week for adults). Exercise has myriad health benefits, including the reduction of stress and improvement of your mental health. You don't have to run a marathon—you don't even have to run. Throw a ball with your kids, go for a walk, ride your bike, lift weights, join a class at the gym . . . do *something* to get your body moving. If you can, get some exercise every day.

Finally, do something for yourself. If you're like the vast majority of people in Western cultures, you're too busy, and you're too stressed out. Take some time to treat yourself to a day at a spa, or even just go out to dinner with your spouse. Do something fun and relaxing—something you don't usually do. You deserve it!

Managing stress is a lifelong endeavor, and there are as many stress-control strategies as there are people, so make sure that you tailor your stress management plan to your particular situation. There are tons of books and websites out there that can help you with stress management, and if you're extremely stressed all the time and don't know what to do about it, you should seriously consider seeing a therapist, as they're very well-equipped to help you with issues like this. You won't regret it.

2.5. 7-Day Schedule

The above steps should be used as follows:

Dietary changes: days 1–7.

General parasite / toxin cleansing: days 1–4.

Candida cleansing: 5–7.

Stress control: days 1–7.

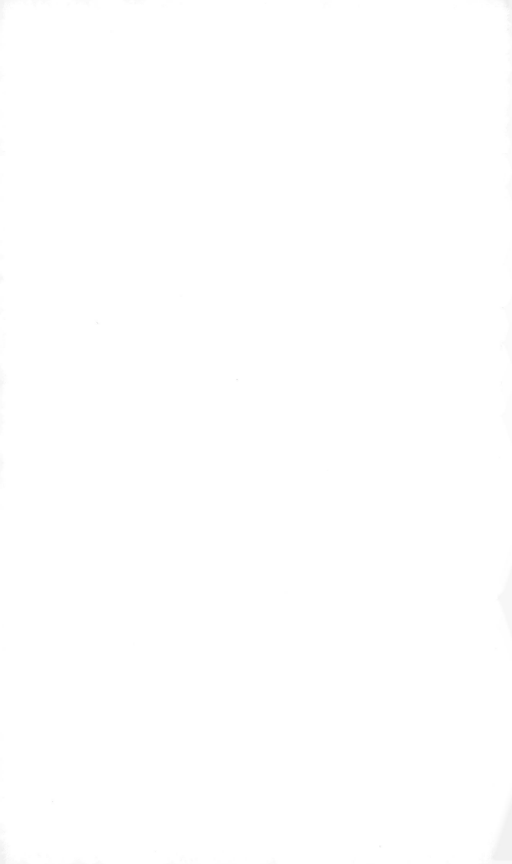

3. Holistic Treatment Plan

Dietary changes are at the heart of natural treatments for GERD. This makes sense, as the primary function of both the esophagus and the stomach have to do with food, so food is likely to play a significant role both in the disorder and in the treatment. Although making dietary changes isn't easy, we have provided you with a guide that will walk you through the key points of how to do it, as well as a sample meal plan and some recipes that will help you get on track.

In addition to dietary changes, however, there are several other lifestyle changes that you will have to make in order to get your body—and your mind—back in balance. Because this is a holistic treatment, it will get at the causes of your GERD, and this will require making many changes to your lifestyle, and this might be difficult; but you'll find that it's worth it.

3.1. Step 1: Dietary Strategies

In making dietary changes, it's important to keep two things in mind: first, a few key points about which foods you should eat, and which you should avoid. Second, there are principles of meal planning that you should observe to make sure that your body is well-prepared to fight off heartburn.

3.1.1 Key Dietary Factors

1. Keep a food diary.

This isn't technically a dietary factor, but it's number one on this list because it's so important. Because everyone is unique, everyone has different triggers for heartburn. Of course, it's best to avoid all of the trigger foods for acid reflux, but if you love spicy food, you'll probably want to make sure that it's one of your triggers before cutting it completely out of your diet.

What's a food diary? It's just like it sounds—a list of the foods you eat, including how much you eat, what time you eat it, and how you feel afterwards. You don't have to spend a lot of time making this extremely detailed—you only need to jot down the information that's most important to helping ease your heartburn. For example, you don't have to write down '100 grams of canned sweet corn'; you can simply write 'medium amount of corn'. Of course, the more detail you can provide, the better, but not everyone has the time to write down all of the details. The time of your meals and snacks is important as well, as you may experience more heartburn at certain times of day (many people find that it's worst at night). This can help you plan your meals accordingly. Finally, write down how the foods you eat make you feel—did that turkey sandwich result in blinding pain in your chest? Or was it just a little? Or maybe none at all? This can help identify the foods that trigger your symptoms.

2. Optimize your fat intake.

Previously, it was stated that delayed emptying of the stomach can be one of the causes of acid reflux. Which foods slow the emptying of the stomach? Those high in fat. By keeping the overall fat in your diet in check, you can help food move through your digestive system at the correct rate, placing less stress on the stomach and the lower esophageal sphincter. What's the correct amount of fat in a daily diet? The answer to that question isn't a simple one, but it's worth discussing.

First, it's important to realize that there are fats that are beneficial, and those that are harmful. You've probably heard about the bad fats, things like trans fats, which are found in partially hydrogenated oils, and saturated fats, which you get from things like red meat, eggs, and dairy products. It's best to keep these to a minimum. Totally cutting them out of your diet often isn't feasible, but you can make an effort to reduce them by replacing items that are high in saturated fat with those that have more unsaturated (healthy) fats. For example, instead of placing a pat of butter into a frying pan to cook with, use a bit of olive oil. Instead of having meat for dinner five nights a week, introduce fish into your diet; the American Heart Association recommends eating fatty fish twice a week.

Second, try to add foods with unsaturated fats to your diet. Low-fat dairy products, beans, and avocados are good sources of these healthy fats, and it's easy to get more of them into your diet (Mexican food, for example, often includes beans and avocados). It's important to keep your overall fat intake in check, though, too—fat should make up around 30% of your total calorie intake for a day. So if you eat an average of 2,200 calories per day, you'd want about 730 of those calories coming from various types of fats. By keeping your fat intake in check and making sure that a good portion of your intake is made up of healthy fats, you'll go a long way toward helping treat your GERD and maintaining a healthy lifestyle (healthy fats are good for your heart, and eating enough of them might help reduce your chances of heart disease). Fortunately, foods that are low in fat are often also low in cholesterol, another substance that can cause problems if you have too much of it.

3. Be careful with protein.

Research on the relationship between protein and acid reflux is inconclusive—some experts say that a high-protein diet contributes to GERD, while others say that this disorder can be treated by consuming a lot of protein. Because the protein in your diet might affect you differently than it could affect someone else, it's best to just keep having protein in moderation. The recommendations for how much of your caloric intake should consist of protein vary quite a bit, but if you're in the 20–25% range, you should be in good shape.

However, because a lot of good sources of protein are high in fat and cholesterol, you should choose your sources wisely. Poultry and fish are good replacements for high-fat meats, and even lean cuts of red meat are better than your standard steak. You're likely going to have to make some trade-offs to make sure you get enough protein. Dairy products, for example, should be consumed in small quantities, but if your daily diet is low in protein, you might want to increase your intake of things like low-fat or Greek yogurt or low-fat cheeses. Eggs are high in protein, but may raise your cholesterol levels. Fortunately, there are some sources of protein that are good all around, like fish, which are also high in healthy fats.

4. Increase fruits, vegetables, and other sources of fiber.

This is actually a couple points in one, but they're all related. First, increase your intake of fruits and vegetables. When has anyone ever said that you eat *too many* fruits and vegetables? Probably never. Well, if you're suffering from acid reflux, they're more important than ever. In addition to myriad general health benefits from fresh (not canned or frozen) fruits and vegetables, they may also help to prevent developing Barrett's esophagus, and they provide a lot of nutrients without overloading you with calories (which is especially important if you're trying to lose weight to combat obesity-related GERD). They're also high in fiber, which is a crucial nutrient for combatting acid reflux and many other gastrointestinal conditions. Fiber helps keep the digestive system clean and functioning correctly, controls blood sugar and prevent ulcers, and keeps harmful toxins from being absorbed by your body. Low-fiber diets have also been associated with conditions like GERD and hiatal hernia, which is a condition that can contribute to acid reflux. To make sure you're getting the most fiber out of your fruits and vegetables, eat them with the skin or peel *on*, instead of peeling them first.

Although increasing fruits and vegetables is important in combatting heartburn, don't get too carried away. Fruits are high in sugar, and some contain acids that might exacerbate the problem you're trying to cure. Citrus fruits, like oranges, lemons, limes, tangerines, and grapefruits, can contribute to an increase in your symptoms, so it's best to stay away from those. Tomatoes are also quite high in acid content, and so should be avoided (as should tomato-based products, like pastes and sauces). Apples, grapes, and bananas are less acidic options, but try them out carefully before adding them to your diet in high amounts. You should also avoid starchy vegetables. Things like potatoes, yams, and corn should be reduced, if not totally cut out, from your diet while you're suffering from gastroesophageal reflux disease. Broccoli and cabbage should also be reduced.

While fruits and vegetables are great sources of fiber, they're not the only ones. Oatmeal and flaxseed provide soluble fiber, while whole grains and nuts are good sources of insoluble fiber—both are important in your diet, and should be consumed on a regular basis. You should be able to reach your recommended fiber intake mostly through fruits and vegetables, but if you're worried about consuming enough (or your doctor tells you to increase your fiber intake), you can supplement with some of the things listed above.

5. Reduce processed sugars.

The average Western diet is absolutely chock full of different kinds of sugar, including sucrose, lactose, fructose, and others. You'll find a surprising amount of added sugar in foods like spaghetti sauce, coffee, instant oatmeal, ketchup, jams, granolas, and dried fruit. If sugar is added to a food, it's almost certainly a highly processed, refined sugar, which may have all sorts of adverse effects on your body if you have too much of it. One man reported reducing his sugar intake because he thought it was inhibiting his ability to concentrate—once he had drastically reduced sugar, he was not only able to concentrate better, but he found that he could breathe more easily and that he had significantly increased energy levels throughout the day.

Processed sugar may have these detrimental effects because it is used differently by the body than naturally occurring sugars, and is more likely to be stored as fat; it places extra stress on your liver and digestive system. It also increases the acidity of your stomach and may promote growth of Candida.

Significantly reducing or eliminating sugar is a great way not only to help your GERD symptoms, but also a way to improve your overall health. Some people believe that processed, white sugar is the underlying cause of most of the prevalent diseases in the Western world, like high blood pressure, diabetes, and heart disease. Regardless of whether or not some of these people are overstating the dangers of sugar, it *is* important to only consume it in moderation. And if you suffer from heartburn, you should definitely make an attempt to reduce it as much as possible to help cure your symptoms. Instead of using refined sugar, use things like raw honey and molasses (and if you absolutely need to use sugar for something, use unrefined, brown sugar).

6. Reduce dairy.

Although the benefits of dairy were mentioned above, it's important to keep your intake moderate. Milk, in addition to being difficult to digest for many people, is also quite acidic, leading to a more acidic environment in the stomach (which, of course, is bad). Because of the sugars in milk, it may also be related to excessive Candida growth in your digestive tract, which may also increase your risk of developing or exacerbating GERD. Many people also point out that dairy cows are given many antibiotics and hormones to keep them healthy and increase their milk production, and these substances might filter down to you, with unknown effects.

If you really like milk (or are concerned about your calcium intake), you can substitute cow's milk with goat's or sheep's milk, especially those which are not pasteurized (the pasteurization alters the sugars that are naturally present in milk). An even better substitute is nut milks, like hazelnut or almond milk, which still allow you to get the milk you crave without the heartburn-promoting side effects. Soy milk is an acceptable substitute, but consuming too much of it may be related to other health problems, so be careful to have it in moderation. Also, if you absolutely can't live without cow's milk, make sure it's non-fat, as the fats in milk cause most of the problems.

7. Reduce spicy foods.

Although scientific studies have shown no proven link between spicy foods and heartburn, you should still be careful. While you're keeping track of what you're eating in your food diary, make notes of how spicy your foods are, and if you find that eating spicy foods triggers your heartburn, cut them out of your diet. Many people find, however, that spicy foods are not among their trigger foods, and that they can keep eating them, so it's worth investigating a bit.

If you want to only cut out some spices, you can start with the ones that are most likely to exacerbate your symptoms—things like red and black pepper, chili, and curry spices. If you decide to remove these from your diet, you can replace them with more mild seasonings, like rosemary and basil. Like with most foods, though, using your food diary is crucial in determining whether or not you should completely cut them out, reduce them, or leave them as they are.

8. Maintain a proper pH level.

The human body functions optimally with an internal pH of 7.0–8.0. Basically, what this means is that the acidity level of your body needs to stay within a certain range to work correctly (in case you're wondering, 7.0–8.0 is somewhere between the acidity of distilled water and sea water; gastric acid is around 1.0, or very acidic, while bleach is around 13.0, or very alkaline). If your body gets out of the acceptable range, you can begin to have a number of problems. For example, if it's too acidic, fungus, yeast, and parasites will be better able to survive in it. If it gets significantly outside of the optimal range, it can cause organ damage. By helping—instead of hindering—your body's pH regulation processes, you can make it less likely that you'll suffer from these acid-alkaline imbalance issues.

So how do you use your diet to help stabilize the pH of your body in the correct range? By eating foods that neutralize acids in your body—foods that are alkaline in their pH. Fortunately, there are plenty of good foods that are alkaline, including carrots, apples, raisins, and almonds, among many others. Some of the minerals that reduce the acidity of your body are calcium, magnesium, potassium, and sodium. While you can't eat *only* alkaline foods, you can try to make sure they make up as much of your diet as possible. You can also avoid acidic foods, like corn, wheat and most other grain products, butter, cheese, most animal proteins, and most medicinal drugs (even ibuprofen and aspirin). This is another place where maintaining a gluten-free diet is helpful. Again, it's clear that you can't cut all of these out, but it's good to be aware of your intake of acidic foods, and to make an effort to keep it moderate.

3.1.1. Meal Planning

You may not realize it, but it's not only the food you eat that affects your heartburn, but also how and when you eat it. For example, if you weaken your lower esophageal sphincter before you eat, you may find that you feel increased pain after eating. So it's important to make sure that you do the right things both before and after your meals to minimize the chances that your GERD will act up. There are several strategies that you can use to optimize your meal planning to reduce your risk of suffering from painful after-effects.

1. Avoid eating large meals.

As was mentioned before, eating too much at one time can put stress on the lower esophageal sphincter, causing it to open and allow gastric acid into the esophagus. By eating smaller, more frequent meals, you can keep the amount of food in your stomach at a reasonable level to avoid this problem.

2. Avoid lying down or exercising after meals.

Both of these things can increase the amount of stomach acid that refluxes back into your esophagus. When you lie down, gravity is no longer helping keep your stomach acids from moving through the lower esophageal sphincter, making it even harder for that muscle to do its job correctly. And exercising causes your body to move blood to your active muscles and away from your digestive system, slowing digestion—it also may contribute to the contents of your stomach moving around and allowing acids into your esophagus. If at all possible, wait at least two hours after a meal to exercise.

3. Combine your foods correctly.

Because some foods are harder for your body to digest, it's important to limit those foods to one serving per meal. Hard-to-digest foods include things like meats, dairy, grains, and starchy foods, and having more than one serving of these foods at one time can both slow digestion and cause the buildup of gas, both of which are detrimental when you're suffering from GERD. Foods that are easier to digest include fruits and non-starchy vegetables. By eating raw vegetables with the hard-to-digest foods listed above, you can help decrease the stress on your digestive system. Similarly, eating fruit by itself or with raw vegetables will help prevent the buildup of gas. By using your food diary, you should be able to discover some food combinations that trigger your symptoms, and you can remove those combinations from your meal planning.

4. Avoid smoking and alcohol before, during, and after meals.

Both smoking and drinking alcohol can weaken the lower esophageal sphincter, and by now, you should know that this is bad. This is especially important around meals that often cause heartburn, like dinner (for most people, anyway; but this varies quite a bit).

5. Eat in a calm, relaxed environment.

Holistic medicine is all about the body as a complete and whole system, which means all of your organs—including your brain and nervous system—are connected. If you're multi-tasking—like eating lunch at your desk at work, or watching TV while you eat breakfast— or if you're stressed, you should take a few minutes before you eat to calm yourself and your environment. The more relaxed you are, and the more focused on the meal that you're eating, the more effective your digestion will be. Some people find that their acid reflux is significantly related to their stress level, and you may find that this is especially true while you're eating. So be mindful about when, where, and how you eat.

3.2. Step 2: Weight Management

As was mentioned previously, being overweight can put you at increased risk of suffering from gastroesophageal reflux disease. If your body mass index (BMI) is above 30, and you are considered to be obese, you put yourself at even greater risk of GERD. Because of this, weight management is an integral part of treating your acid reflux, or reducing your risk of developing it. If you keep your body at the proper weight, you'll be doing yourself a huge favor, even beyond reducing your likelihood of suffering from acid reflux.

This is because obesity is at the heart of many other disorders and conditions that are common in the Western world (and are often attributable to the sub-optimal diet that is common in our culture), including Type 2 diabetes, various heart diseases, liver problems, and cancer. Exactly how being overweight is linked to these conditions isn't always clear, but if there's one thing that health professionals all around the world agree upon, it's that managing your weight is crucial to managing your health.

By following the dietary guidelines in the previous section, you'll be part of the way to ensuring that you maintain a healthy weight. Optimizing your fat intake, increasing fruits and vegetables, and reducing processed sugar and dairy will all help you eat the right number of calories in a day. However, losing weight isn't just about eating the right foods. It's also about eating the right *amount* of food, which can be much more difficult. And it's about a lot of other

44

things, too. Strategies for losing weight are as varied as they are common, but here are four easy steps you can take to regulate your food intake. Obviously, if you are overweight (especially if you're significantly overweight), you should speak with your doctor about healthy ways to lose weight and improve your health.

1. Adopt strategies to keep your calorie intake under control.

Obviously, the issue at the core of being overweight is that you consume more calories than you burn on a daily basis. It doesn't even have to be a lot—even if it's only a couple pounds a year, it adds up pretty quickly. Think about it: if you add two pounds every year, in ten years, you'll be twenty pounds heavier than you are right now. That sounds like a long time, but it'll be here before you know it. So adopting strategies that will help you keep your calorie count in the correct range is crucial. The first strategy, and possibly best one, is to start a food journal. I've already recommended keeping a food log to discover your heartburn trigger foods, but this log can also have the added benefit of helping you keep track of when you eat more than you should. If you really want to lose weight, I highly recommend using something tailor-made for the purpose. There are plenty of food journals out there that will help you keep track of daily calorie count, and lately there have been an increasing number of apps for your computer (both web-based and otherwise), as well as your iPhone, iPad, or Android device. Just run a search in the app store and you'll see tons of options, some of which are free (LoseIt is a favorite of mine). Try one out and see what you think. It'll seem like a ton of work at first, but it gets a lot easier.

One of the simplest methods for keeping your caloric intake down is to use smaller dishes. This sounds a bit ridiculous, but by using a smaller plate, you're forced to take smaller portions—give it a shot, and you'll see what I mean.

2. Get rid of unhealthy foods.

One of the best ways to make your diet more amenable to weight loss is to remove unhealthy foods from your kitchen. If you're serious about losing weight as soon as possible, do it right now. Toss the cookies, the candies, and the frozen pizza. If weight loss is less of an immediate concern for you, keep these in moderation, but *don't buy them* next time you're at the grocery store. If you don't buy a certain food, you won't be able to eat it at home (of course, you'll need to use more self-control at the grocery store and when you go out, but you have to start somewhere). Fill your cart with lots of fresh produce and lean sources of protein. If you're craving something salty, go with some lightly salted mixed nuts to get the nutrients they offer without consuming lots of extra processed sugar.

3. Tell other people you're trying to lose weight.

Losing weight on your own, without anybody's help, is really difficult. Some people are embarrassed about their weight, and I understand this, but you have to resist the temptation to keep your weight loss efforts a secret. Tell your family members, your friends, and your co-workers. Tell them to keep you accountable—if they see you grabbing a donut in the conference room, or a bowl of ice cream out of the freezer, you want them to remind you that you should be having healthier options. Finding someone to join you in your weight loss efforts is even better—you can count calories together, exercise together, and celebrate together when you've reached your goals. I can't over-state the importance of this. You don't have to take all of this on by yourself, and you shouldn't try to.

4. Make exercise a habit.

This is a crucial point, and it requires serious lifestyle modification. Most people aren't getting enough exercise, and it's hard to change the habits that you've developed over many years of sedentary (or mostly sedentary) living. But now is the time to put the past behind you and make a change—if you're really committed to losing weight and managing your GERD, exercise is an invaluable tool. Not only does it burn a lot of calories, establishing the crucial calorie deficit that you need (by creating a calorie deficit of 500 calories each day, you'll lose 1 pound per week), but it's also very beneficial for stress control, which will also help your heartburn.

So how do you make exercise a habit? This depends on a lot on you and your lifestyle, but finding an exercise partner is a good first step. Your spouse, a sibling, a friend, a co-worker . . . anyone who will commit to exercising with you at least a couple times a week (if you're trying to lose weight, exercising often is critical; aim for three to four days every week, in addition to your dietary efforts). Meet to go for a walk, or meet at the gym to lift weights or attend a fitness class, or just throw a ball around in the yard. Join a community softball team, or pick up a new activity, like tennis. If you used to play a sport in college, and you miss it, it's likely that there's a group somewhere near you that also plays that sport on a casual, non-competitive basis.

Another great way to make exercise a habit is to put it on your calendar. Most people have some sort of central calendar now, whether on their phone, on their computer, or stored online, like with Google Calendar or Apple's iCal. Plan out your exercise schedule for the next week or two, and put it on your calendar so you don't forget. Set up really annoying alarms if you have to (especially if you're going to be exercising early in the morning, before work). If you have an exercise partner, share your calendar events so neither of you forgets. You'd be surprised at how motivated you are if your calendar tells you that you have to exercise (exactly what that says about us as a society and how highly we regard our electronic devices, I'm not sure). Another good thing you can do with a calendar is record your daily weight on it. Weigh yourself in the morning, before you eat, and note the results. Also keep your goal weight on the calendar—if you're approaching your goal date, and you haven't quite made it to your goal weight yet, you'll be surprised at how motivated you are to get there when you see it on your calendar.

Finally, take little steps. If you're going to make exercise a part of your daily life, it's best to incorporate it in every way you can. Take the stairs instead of the escalator; park further away from the grocery store and walk; bike to the grocery store if you only need a couple things and can fit them in a backpack; get up and go for a 15-minute walk a few times a day while you're at work. All of these little things add up, and will help you create a calorie deficit on a regular basis. You don't have to go on a long run or play a 2-hour game of basketball to do it (although, obviously, that'll get you there faster).

Weight management isn't something that's easy, and it's very rarely a steady and consistent process. You'll be at one weight one day, a couple pounds lighter the next week, a few heavier the week after that, several pounds lighter the following week, and just under where you started the next week. Remember that it's a long-term commitment that is crucial for your health, both related to GERD and in general. It's tough, but it's worth it. Don't get discouraged, and keep it up!

3.3. Step 3: Detox / Parasite Cleanse

An important part of treating your acid reflux disease is periodically cleansing your gastrointestinal tract. By ridding your body of toxins, you lessen the strain on your vital organs and allow for those toxins to be safely flushed out of your system—this is crucial in supporting your acid reflux treatment, as a high toxin load in your body will contribute to many problems, including GERD. How often you go through a cleansing period is up to you, and depends greatly on the type of cleanse. What's outlined here is a non-fasting cleanse, and can be maintained easily for longer than can a fasting cleanse, such as a juice fast. Some experts recommend juice fasting, but if you are going to conduct something like this, you should speak with your doctor or a medical professional who understands the benefits, risks, and best practices of juice fasting.

The first thing to know about cleansing is that it's not just a dietary activity, but a lifestyle that you must adopt for the time that you are fasting. Most of the things that I will recommend are good things to keep in mind all the time, but they are especially important during a cleansing period.

Being mentally committed to your cleanse is of utmost importance. In addition to your body, you must cleanse your mind. Your cleansing period should be as low-stress as possible—obviously, you can only remove so much stress from your life, but you should take extra steps to ensure that you can handle your stressors as best as possible during this period. Perform extra meditation sessions, engage in extra (gentle) activity, and remove as many distractors from your life as you can. If you don't need your cell phone for a period of time, turn it off. Reduce the amount of time you spend in front of a computer screen or the TV (read a book instead). All of these things will help your mind reach the right state during the cleanse, which is crucial for your body to perform at its best.

Getting enough sleep is also important during the cleanse. Obviously, it's always important, but when you're asleep, your body can heal itself, and this is the point of a cleanse. By giving your body the time it needs to expel toxins and heal the damage they've done, you'll be setting yourself up for success. Try to get at least 8 hours every night; if you absolutely can't do that during the week, try to catch up on the weekends. Sleep a bit during the day if you need to. Make sure to listen to your body, especially when it's telling you that it needs extra rest (which it might during this time).

Finally, practice mindfulness. Exactly what mindfulness means differs between people, but what should be emphasized here is that you need to be in close connection with your body. Your body is constantly communicating with you, and making sure that you're listening is extremely important during a cleanse. Your body may tell you to rest, or that it needs more exercise, or that the specifics of your cleanse diet aren't working for you, in which case you should alter it a bit. But remember that what you *think* your body is telling you isn't always necessarily correct, so be extra mindful of what you need. Many people *think* that their body is telling them to eat a big bacon cheeseburger . . . but that's pretty unlikely. Food cravings and real hunger are quite different, and it's good to keep that difference in mind during the cleanse.

Now, onto the actual dietary guidelines for the cleanse. You'll notice that many of these foods are the ones that were recommended previously for dealing with GERD. You may also notice that several of the recommended foods are ones that you should avoid while treating your heartburn, and you may think this is contradictory. Unfortunately, if you were to stick with only foods that were renowned for their cleansing abilities *and* beneficial for heartburn, you'd have a very small choice of foods. Because of this, I encourage you to add—in very small amounts—a bit of variety in your cleansing foods. Be very aware of which ones cause increased heartburn and remove them from your diet as soon as possible. You may find that there are some foods that don't affect you as much as you expected, though, and feel alright about leaving them in. This is okay, too. As with most things, the most important piece of advice to be offered is that you should listen to your body. With that said, here are the guidelines.

1. Eat a lot of green vegetables.

You should always be eating a lot of green vegetables, but during a cleanse, you need to step it up. Get lots of leafy vegetables like kale, collards, and spinach, but also include broccoli, avocado, mustard greens, dandelion roots, and artichokes. Raw vegetables are best, but if it's easier for you, feel free to give them a light steam first. A cleansing diet is a great time to try a lot of salads, and to snack on vegetables, to increase your intake.

2. Add cleansing fruits.

Certain fruits are great for cleansing your digestive system. Things like apples, grapefruit, limes, and lemons are among the best. Obviously, these are quite acidic, so you should only have them in moderation—and if they make your heartburn worse, you can skip them all together. Try to get at least a few in, though, when you can.

3. Add more vegetables.

If you thought you couldn't eat any more vegetables after adding the leafy green ones, think again. You should also increase your intake of carrots, beets, onions, and cabbage. The reason for adding so many vegetables is that they are high in insoluble fiber, which is one of the best nutrients for cleaning out your system, as well as a large amount of micronutrients—vitamins, minerals, flavonoids, and other things like that—that are difficult to get from other sources. So load up on those vegetables!

4. Have a few whole grains.

Whether you've gone gluten-free or not, adding a small-to-moderate amount of whole grains to your diet during this time will be beneficial. Brown rice, wild rice, sorghum, millet, and buckwheat are all good choices here. Pseudograins like quinoa and amaranth are also acceptable, though slightly less beneficial. Whole grains will provide you with crucial soluble fiber, as well as B vitamins.

5. Season with garlic.

Although garlic can be one of the trigger foods for heartburn, it is also known as a very powerful cleansing agent. Before adding too much to your diet, make sure that it doesn't upset your system too much by trying just a little bit at a time (adding a few chopped garlic cloves to a stir fry is a great way to try this out). If you can handle it, season your savory meals with garlic so you can get the cleansing benefits.

6. Drink green tea.

Green tea has long been known as one of the most beneficial beverages. Of course, you have to make a trade here between a harsh, caffeinated beverage and your cleansing diet (it's never simple, is it?). In addition to providing a diuretic effect—which is not always good, but certainly helps you remove toxins from your system—it contains a huge number of anti-oxidants, which may help to prevent several conditions, possibly including cancer.

As you can see, you're going to have to do some experimentation with your cleansing foods, as a lot of them are potential trigger foods. Don't compromise your GERD diet for the cleanse; instead, find the optimal foods that allow you to keep your heartburn under control while also helping your body rid itself of toxins. And remember: when in doubt, talk to your doctor.

3.4. Step 4: Immune / Digestive / Anti-Candida Supplements

Although adopting a proper diet will help you get the nutrients you need, it doesn't provide *everything* that you need. Because of the makeup of our diets, the way our bodies work, and how food is grown and processed, supplementing your diet with various substances is of high importance. If you've paid attention to the news (especially health-related news) over the past decade or so, you've probably heard about a lot of different supplements; some that have been shown to be beneficial, and some that have been shown to be hoaxes. How can you tell the difference? To be completely honest, it can be difficult at times. But sticking with tried-and-true supplements will help keep you from ingesting harmful substances. Of course, supplementing your diet with things like vitamin complexes, multi-vitamins, and essential fatty acids is something that you should discuss with your doctor, especially if you have any health conditions or are currently on any medications. In addition to this, your doctor can help you keep up on the latest research on dietary supplements.

That said, here is a list of four supplements that you can feel confident about taking on a regular basis. All of them will help in some way or another with your reflux disease, and most of them will also have benefits for your general health. Remember that supplements are no replacement for a healthy diet, but serve the function that's in their name—supplementing.

1. Essential fatty acids.

You've probably heard about essential fatty acids, even if you're not aware of it. Omega-3s, Omega-6s, and Omega-9s are all types of essential fatty acids that abound in the body, and maintaining a proper balance of these substances is crucial in managing inflammation (which is important when you're dealing with acid reflux). Unfortunately, the typical Western diet promotes a bodily environment that is high in Omega-6 and Omega-9 acids, and deficient in Omega-3s, which are found in cold-water fish (like herring, mackerel, salmon, swordfish, cod, catfish, and many others), as well as some plants, including kiwi, flax, lingonberry, and canola. To make a long, scientific story short, you probably aren't getting enough Omega-3s, and this is likely to cause an excess of inflammation in your body, which is bad. In addition to consuming more foods that contain Omega-3s (especially cold-water fish), you should be supplementing your diet with Omega-3. This is often found in fish oil pills, but you may also be able to find flaxseed- or algae-derived oils. There are many different supplements to choose from, each of which has its own special composition. Asking your doctor for a recommendation is the best way to go here.

2. Magnesium.

In addition to being a natural antacid, magnesium helps the muscles in your body relax. After reading about the lower esophageal sphincter and how a lack of muscle tone in this important muscle can contribute to heartburn, this may seem like a bad idea. However, spasms in the muscles of your stomach can be a major contributor to acid reflux, and so taking magnesium to help prevent these spasms can be hugely helpful.

3. Digestive enzymes.

Because digestion is at the heart of GERD and related issues, it makes sense to do whatever you can to help make sure that your body is digesting properly. In addition to adjusting your eating habits, one of the best things you can do to this end is to supplement your diet with digestive enzymes, including protease, amylase, cellulase, and lactase. These enzymes are already present in your body, but by ensuring that they're present in the right quantities, you can significantly assist your body in maintaining proper digestion. There are many different supplements with digestive enzymes, but natural ones like papaya enzymes and orange peel extract are some of the best sources. Of course, talking to your doctor about which enzymes you may need to supplement with is crucial, and you can also consult trained professionals at health food stores, who might be able to help you choose the proper supplement.

4. Anti-Candida supplements.

As was mentioned in the emergency 7-day treatment, killing off Candida is a crucial step in allowing your body to heal itself and return to its normal functions. Although starving Candida by cutting sugar out of your diet is a viable strategy, not everyone is willing (or able) to do this. Another—not quite as good, but still effective—strategy is to use anti-Candida supplements to help get it under control. There are many different supplements that are made to target Candida, and they include things like black walnut, oregano oil, cloves, caprylic acid, and wormwood. They often have names like SporeGone and Candigest. Take one of these on a regular basis during the beginning of your treatment, but don't rely on it forever; your body is equipped with the proper immune functions to keep Candida under control once your diet has improved.

It's important to remember that the vast majority of your nutrients should be provided by a healthy, balanced, and focused diet. However, many factors go into proper nutrient intake, and unless you grow all of your own food, at least some of the nutrients will be lost in the processing, shipment, or storage. Because of this, supplementing your diet is an important step in dealing with your acid reflux disease.

3.5. Step 5: Boost Beneficial Bacteria

The human body is host to billions of bacteria and other tiny organisms, the vast majority of which will remain totally unnoticed throughout the entirety of your life. Just like Candida, however, sometimes these organisms require some intervention to remain in proper balance. Although the list of bacteria and their functions is far too long to reproduce here, it's safe to say that a huge number of digestive disorders can be caused or exacerbated by an imbalance of these bacteria. Fortunately, reducing the acidity of your body is a good first step in supporting the growth of these beneficial organisms (see part 1 of chapter 3, section 1 for more information on maintaining a proper pH level in your body), and maintaining a healthy and balanced diet also goes a long way. But again, the way in which the Western world manages its food sources and supply often leaves it without some of the crucial nutrients that we need.

Luckily, there are many options for supplementation that will help you restore the bacteria in your digestive tract to the proper levels. These probiotics, as they are known, will help you maintain the proper organisms in your digestive system, and in this way, help optimize your digestion. Although there are many different probiotics, the two you should focus on are acidophilus and lacto bifidus. There are many different probiotic supplements that contain these, but it's important to find one that is labeled as a whole food probiotic, as it will have the most beneficial effect.

In addition to supplementing with probiotics, you should also be consuming a large number of prebiotic foods, which provide the nutrients that will help the bacteria in your digestive system thrive once they have established themselves. As mentioned previously, prebiotic foods include tomatoes, onions, bananas, garlic, and asparagus. The combination of probiotic supplements and prebiotic foods will keep the beneficial bacteria in your system healthy and at the proper levels.

3.6. Step 6: Stress Control

The final step in the holistic treatment plan is stress control. As the body is one big, integrated system, your mind can have a strong effect on your GERD symptoms (and most other parts of your physical body, as well, but that won't be addressed here). Being in a state of stress, especially for long periods of time, can have harmful effects that are both mental and physical, and one common physical symptom of prolonged exposure to stress is heartburn. Of course, there are many factors that contribute to acid reflux disease, but by treating as many of the underlying causes as possible, you will cure yourself more completely and gain more general health benefits on the side. Stress control is a lifelong exercise that may take years to perfect and integrate into your daily lifestyle, but there are a few methods that you can start with to get the ball rolling. If these methods don't work for you, there are dozens more—search the internet, talk to your doctor, or see a therapist to get more information on alternative strategies to the four presented here.

1. Identify your stressors.

What stresses you out? Do you know the answer immediately upon reading that question, or do you need a moment to think about it? Sometimes there are obvious causes (heartburn can be not only a symptom of stress, but also a *cause* of stress), but sometimes it's harder to know what's taking a toll on your mental health. Sit down in a quiet place and write about it. Write down things that are causing you stress, even if it's just a little bit. Once you're done, look over your list and think about what you can do to help manage the stress coming from each one. Even better than this is to keep a stress journal, in which you write down when you feel stress, what causes it, how it makes you feel, and what you did about it. This can be an extremely insightful activity, and help you get well on your way to successfully managing your stress.

2. Take time for yourself.

This is one of the hardest things for people to do, especially in modern, Western, professional cultures. Do you always have your cell phone on and your e-mail open? Do you bring work home with you? Do you work on the weekends? These are all things that contribute to work-related stress. By adding this to a family life (if you're a parent, you'll really understand this), a social life, and a romantic life (with a spouse or any sort of partner), you're putting yourself at a big disadvantage when it comes to stress. While most of these things are rewarding, and many are enjoyable, if you do them constantly without giving yourself a chance to rest, you're going to get overwhelmed and stressed out. By taking time out for yourself, you'll let your mind effectively catch its breath, and you'll be refreshed enough to deal with all of the stressors of life without getting overwhelmed.

So what can you do about it? Make time for yourself. Not for you and your spouse, or you and your family, or you and your friends; just for *you*. It's going to seem difficult at first. You might even feel a bit selfish. But once you've started making a habit of this, you'll realize the immense value of the practice. Choosing the right thing to do for yourself is up to you. If going down to a local coffee shop and reading a book is what you need, then go for it. Put a couple hours on your calendar, and don't change them unless you absolutely have to— and then enjoy some relaxing time with a book. If you want to spend a Saturday at a spa, getting a massage, a manicure, and a facial, do it. Schedule it now. Sometimes all you need is 30 minutes to go for a walk and be silent. Only you know exactly what you need, so take a little time to think about it, and do it. You'll be amazed at how much better you feel. To really help you manage your stress, set aside some time every day—even if it's just for something like a bath or a walk.

And finally, remember that having fun is a crucially important part of your life! Do fun and goofy things every once in a while, even if it feels a little strange at first. Sarah Jio, a writer for Vitamin G, once wrote that singing helped her blow off steam. Everyone needs levity and frivolity in their lives, especially if they're stressed out!

3. Get enough sleep.

This is often overlooked, especially if you're someone who has a lot to do all the time. Intuitively, you'd think that sleeping a little less would allow you to get more done and leave you with fewer stressors. However, it doesn't work that way. Most people who have tried this will tell you one of two things: either that you eventually crash really hard and become ill, or that no matter how much you get done, there's still more to do. This is an unfortunate fact of life—you just can't do it all. So make sure that you're getting eight hours of sleep every night to make sure that you have the energy and mental clarity to deal with your day.

Research shows that sleep can have a huge effect on your life, and not getting enough of it is never going to be helpful. If you can't sleep in a little later, go to bed a little earlier. If you end up not sleeping enough during the week, sleep in an extra hour on Saturday. If you still don't feel caught up, take an afternoon nap. Many people feel lazy if they sleep in or take a nap, but it's important to remember that sleep is absolutely crucial to proper functioning, and will go a long way in helping you manage your stress (and, therefore, your GERD).

4. Learn to say no.

This is the most important, and the most difficult, stress management technique for most people. It's a hard thing to come to terms with, but many of the things that you have to do are ones that you agreed to, when you could've said no, but you said yes. You could've declined to host this month's book club, but you're happy to help out. You could've told your boss that you, in fact, *didn't* have time to take on an extra project. If you start paying close attention, you'll realize that there are hundreds of little things that you've agreed to do. And usually, that's fine. But sometimes they add up to a really stressful level, and you need to start saying no. If you feel bad just telling someone 'no', you can tell them that you're treating your acid reflux disease by managing your time and stress. Or don't tell them anything at all—how you handle these situations is up to you, but remember that taking care of yourself will make you fresher, happier, and better able to handle your life and enjoy the things that you like to do. It's a win-win situation, and if you think about it, you'll realize that when you say no to something, you're not going to cause serious difficulties for anyone, or experience anything so dramatic as a falling out or a big fight. It's pretty unlikely that being honest about the time you have at work will result in your losing your job. Remember that just about everyone benefits from your increased ability to manage your stress—and say no.

This is a very short list, but I encourage you to seek out other methods of stress relief and stress management. Not only for your GERD, but for your general physical and mental health.

4. Other Alternative Treatments

In addition to the above listed emergency 7-day plan and the holistic treatment plan, there are a few other ways that you can ease your GERD symptoms and help address the causes. Some people find these alternative treatments to be very effective, while others find that they don't help at all. It depends totally on your symptoms and your body. If you feel that you could use an extra boost in your treatment, I encourage you to look into some of these options and make enquiries with local providers to see what they can offer you.

4.1. Massage

There are many different types of massage, and different providers are able to target different problems. Obviously, a masseuse that specializes in loosening stress-clenched muscles isn't going to do your digestive issues much good (though it may help a lot to reduce your stress, which will certainly be beneficial). Some providers, however, are practitioners of holistic medicine, and can target specific areas of your body that require stimulation to help your digestive system perform optimally.

Digestive massage is a great choice, as it helps move food through your digestive system at the proper speed (one of the problems that may contribute to GERD is slow movement of food due to slow muscles in the stomach), and will stimulate the stomach and intestines to aid proper digestion. Lymph drainage massage may also help your acid reflux, as the buildup of toxins (such as from Candida overgrowth) can disrupt the proper flow of lymph throughout your body, resulting in imbalances that can result in a worsening of symptoms. By keeping your lymph flowing correctly, you will better be able to flush toxins out of your system. Finally, gland and organ massage may also help with the proper flow of substances (like lymph and hormones) throughout your body, which will also help you expel toxins. Even myofascial release techniques, which are generally used for tight muscles, can have an effect—one student of massage therapy reported that her sister had tried many different medications, but couldn't get rid of her heartburn; once she started undergoing regular massage therapy, her GERD got a lot better.

4.2. Acupuncture

Acupuncture, like massage, is used to treat many different types of issues. It has been practiced for several centuries, primarily in Chinese medicine, with the goal of reinstating the body's natural energy flow; if this energy flow is disrupted, many symptoms can result, including heartburn. Some modern practitioners also practice a similar technique called dry-needling, which is focused more on ameliorating muscular pain, but you may also be able to find someone familiar with the techniques that would be willing to help you with acid reflux. Acupuncture is also sometimes aided by electrical stimulation through the inserted needles, which further affects the energy flow of the body and helps to restore it to its natural state. If you are interested in this treatment method, talk to several acupuncturists in your area to see which ones are best equipped to treat GERD and other digestive disorders.

4.3. Homeopathy and aromatherapy

Two other alternative strategies that are used to combat GERD are aromatherapy, which uses essential oils, and homeopathy, which involves the exposure of the body to certain toxins that are already present in the body in an effort to familiarize your defenses with the toxin and better train them to deal with it. There are, of course, other alternatives medicines that may help you in your fight against acid reflux disease—talk to your doctor or a trained and certified therapy provider to discuss the best options for you.

45 Delicious Acid Reflux Friendly Recipes

BREAKFAST

1. 100% Buckwheat Pancakes

Servings: 2-3
Serving size: 2 pancakes
Total time: 30 minutes

Nutrition Facts

Serving Size 357 g

Amount Per Serving

Calories 594	Calories from Fat 135

	% Daily Value*
Total Fat 15.0g	**23%**
Saturated Fat 6.2g	**31%**
Trans Fat 0.0g	
Cholesterol 116mg	**39%**
Sodium 1059mg	**44%**
Total Carbohydrates 101.6g	**34%**
Dietary Fiber 9.4g	**38%**
Sugars 39.5g	
Protein 20.8g	

Vitamin A 7%	•	Vitamin C 6%
Calcium 29%	•	Iron 26%

Nutrition Grade B
* Based on a 2000 calorie diet

Ingredients

- 1 teaspoon canola oil
- 1 large egg (optional)
- 1 1/2 cup low-fat buttermilk
- 1 1/2 cup buckwheat flour

65

- 1/8 teaspoon salt
- 3 tablespoon unrefined brown sugar
- 1 teaspoon baking soda
- 3 teaspoon unsalted butter (or Fat-Free Buttermilk)
- 2 Tablespoon maple syrup (organic pure maple syrup is best) or Jam
- ¼ cup frozen blueberries

Directions

1. In a large bowl, whisk together the buckwheat flour, salt, sugar, and baking soda. Slowly blend in the melted butter until smooth.
2. Whisk the egg and mix into buttermilk. Blend egg mixture into the buckwheat batter gently. For a more light and fluffy pancake, let the batter sit for 10-15 minutes or overnight.
3. Melt one teaspoon of the butter onto a hot griddle or frying pan and then spoon about 1/3 cup of batter to form pancakes. Flip the pancakes over once bubbles form and burst on top of them, then cook the other side until golden brown.
4. Serve hot, topped with the additional butter, maple syrup or jam, and frozen blueberries.

2. Fruit-and-Nut Power Bars

Servings: 8
Serving size: 1 bar
Total time: 30 minutes
Note: This recipe makes good leftovers.

Nutrition Facts

Serving Size 49 g

Amount Per Serving

Calories 107	Calories from Fat 47

	% Daily Value*
Total Fat 5.2g	8%
Saturated Fat 0.6g	3%
Trans Fat 0.0g	
Cholesterol 0mg	0%
Sodium 75mg	3%
Total Carbohydrates 14.6g	5%
Dietary Fiber 2.0g	8%
Sugars 11.6g	
Protein 2.7g	

Vitamin A 5%	•	Vitamin C 3%
Calcium 2%	•	Iron 6%

Nutrition Grade B
* Based on a 2000 calorie diet

Ingredients

- 1/2 cup whole Medjool dates (about 5), halved and pitted
- 1/4 cup dried plums (prunes)
- 1/2 cup dried apricots
- 1 cup whole raw almonds
- 1/4 teaspoon salt
- 1/4 cup raw pumpkin seeds
- 1/4 cup raw sunflower seeds
- 1 teaspoon or coconut oil or olive oil

Directions

1. Preheat oven to 325°.
2. In a food processor, pulse only the nuts and salt until coarsely chopped but still chunky. Place nuts into a mixing bowl. Pour the dates, dried apricots, and dried plums into the food processor and pulse a few times until it makes a paste. Add pumpkin seeds and sunflower seeds, pulsing a few times. Combine the date mixture to the nuts.

3. Grease a baking sheet with coconut oil. Scoop mixture onto the greased baking sheet. Using a rolling pin, roll out the mixture to your desired thickness (preferably 1/2 in).
4. Cut the rolled out mixture into a log shape and desired width (preferably about 1 3/4 in. wide).
5. Bake until center is firm and edges are golden, about 25 minutes. Let cool and store in an airtight container for up to 4 days.

3. Flaxseed and Pumpkin Bread

Servings: 4
Serving size: 1 medium bowl
Total time: 35-45 minutes

Nutrition Facts

Serving Size 109 g

Amount Per Serving	
Calories 266	Calories from Fat 167
	% Daily Value*
Total Fat 18.6g	**29%**
Saturated Fat 4.3g	**21%**
Trans Fat 0.0g	
Cholesterol 0mg	**0%**
Sodium 290mg	**12%**
Total Carbohydrates 17.6g	**6%**
Dietary Fiber 6.2g	**25%**
Sugars 9.0g	
Protein 7.8g	

Vitamin A 22%	•	Vitamin C 3%
Calcium 4%	•	Iron 3%

Nutrition Grade C
* Based on a 2000 calorie diet

Ingredients
- 1 cup blanched almond flour
- ½ teaspoon baking soda
- 1 tablespoon ground cinnamon
- 1 teaspoon ground nutmeg
- ½ teaspoon ground cloves
- ¼ teaspoon sea salt
- ½ cup roasted pumpkin, mashed
- 2 tablespoons raw honey
- ¼ teaspoon stevia (or unrefined brown sugar)

- 3 tablespoons ground flaxseeds
- 1/2 cup water
- 1 tablespoon coconut oil

Directions
1. Preheat oven to 350 degrees F. Grease a mini loaf pan (about 8x4 inch) with coconut oil.
2. In a medium bowl, stir together ground flaxseeds and water until thick. Set aside. In a separate bowl, combine almond flour, baking soda, salt, cinnamon, nutmeg, and cloves; mix well. Add pumpkin, flaxseed mixture, honey, and stevia. Blend well.
3. Pour batter into the loaf pan and bake for 35-45 minutes. Insert a toothpick into the center of the loaf; if it comes out clean it's done, else return the loaf to the oven and bake for a few more minutes.

4. Nutmeg-Maple French Toast
Servings: 4
Serving Size: 1 slice
Total time: 30 minutes

Nutrition Facts

Serving Size 92 g

Amount Per Serving

Calories 164	Calories from Fat 15
	% Daily Value*
Total Fat 1.7g	**3%**
Cholesterol 2mg	**1%**
Sodium 338mg	**14%**
Total Carbohydrates 28.8g	**10%**
Dietary Fiber 1.0g	**4%**
Sugars 7.2g	
Protein 7.6g	

Vitamin A 4%	•	Vitamin C 0%
Calcium 3%	•	Iron 9%

Nutrition Grade B-
* Based on a 2000 calorie diet

Ingredients
- 6 Tablespoon egg substitute
- 2 teaspoon Splenda or stevia
- 6 Tablespoon 2% milk

- 1/4 teaspoon ground nutmeg
- 1/2 teaspoon pure vanilla extract
- 1/8 teaspoon salt
- 4 thick slices gluten free sourdough bread (or challah bread)
- 1 teaspoon low-fat unsalted butter (per serving)
- 1 Tablespoon pure maple syrup (per serving)

Directions

1. In a large mixing bowl, whisk together, Splenda, ground nutmeg, and salt. Mix in the milk and vanilla, and then the egg substitute.
2. Heat a non-stick griddle or frying pan over medium-high heat. Gently dunk and turn each slice of bread into the egg mixture until it is well coated and slightly soaked.
3. Reduce heat to medium. Place the 4 slices of soaked bread on the griddle and cook for about 3 – 4 minutes on both sides until golden brown.
4. Serve hot and top each toast with one teaspoon of butter and one tablespoon pure maple syrup.

5. Pecan Cinnamon Rolls

Servings: 18
Serving size: 1 roll
Total time: 1 hour, 20 minutes

Nutrition Facts

Serving Size 80 g

Amount Per Serving

Calories 224   Calories from Fat 120

% Daily Value*

Total Fat 13.3g	**21%**
Saturated Fat 6.5g	**32%**
Trans Fat 0.0g	
Cholesterol 36mg	**12%**
Sodium 248mg	**10%**
Total Carbohydrates 25.8g	**9%**
Dietary Fiber 1.4g	**6%**
Sugars 20.3g	
Protein 2.0g	

Vitamin A 6%   •   Vitamin C 0%
Calcium 3%   •   Iron 3%

Nutrition Grade D

* Based on a 2000 calorie diet

Ingredients

Dough:

- 1/4 cup warm water (110 degrees F)
- 1/4 cup low-fat butter, melted
- 1/2 (3.4 ounce) package instant vanilla pudding mix
- 1 cup warm milk
- 1 egg, room temperature
- 1 tablespoon unrefined brown sugar
- 1/2 teaspoon salt
- 4 cups gluten-free bread flour
- 1 (0.25 ounce) package active dry yeast

Cinnamon Filling:

- 1/4 cup low-fat butter, softened
- 1 cup unrefined brown sugar
- 4 teaspoons ground cinnamon
- 3/4 cup chopped pecans

Butter Frosting:

- 1/2 (8 ounce) package low-fat cream cheese, softened (room temperature)

- 1/4 cup low-fat butter, softened (room temperature)
- 1 cup unrefined brown sugar
- 1/2 teaspoon vanilla extract
- 1 1/2 teaspoons low-fat milk

Directions
1. Butter a 9 x 13 x 2-inch baking pan; set aside.
2. In a large mixing bowl, combine butter, vanilla pudding mix, milk, sugar, and salt. Dissolve the yeast in the warm water in a separate bowl. Let rest for 5 minutes. Add egg, 2 cups flour and the yeast mixture. Beat until smooth. Mix in remaining flour by adding 1 cup at a time until soft dough forms.
3. (If using a bread machine, place dough ingredients in the pan and set machine to Dough cycle; press Start. When the machine has completed the dough cycle, remove dough from pan.)
4. Using a rolling pin, roll and stretch dough on a lightly floured surface until smooth and elastic (about 4 to 6 minutes) to form an approximately 15 x 24-inch rectangle.
5. Spread the softened butter over the top of the dough using a spatula or pastry brush. Combine and sprinkle the cinnamon filling mixture over dough.
6. Beginning with long edge, roll up dough. Slice into 16 one inch slices and place in 9x13 buttered pan. Cover and let them rise for 45 minutes until doubled. Meanwhile, preheat oven to 350 degrees F (175 degrees C).
7. Bake in preheated oven for approximately 15 to 20 minutes until they are a light golden brown. Combine butter frosting ingredients. Remove rolls from oven and top with frosting.

To Freeze Unbaked Rolls: Cover unbaked cinnamon rolls with plastic wrap. Wrap tightly with heavy-duty foil. Store in freezer up to 2 months.

To Prepare Frozen Unbaked Rolls: Remove rolls from freezer. Allow to thaw completely and rise at room temperature for 30 minutes. Uncover and bake at 350° for 20 minutes or until browned.

6. Walnut Carrot Muffins

Servings: 6
Serving size: 1 muffin
Total time: 30 Minutes

Nutrition Facts

Serving Size 127 g

Amount Per Serving

Calories 284	Calories from Fat 68
	% Daily Value*
Total Fat 7.6g	**12%**
Saturated Fat 0.6g	**3%**
Trans Fat 0.0g	
Cholesterol 1mg	**0%**
Sodium 221mg	**9%**
Total Carbohydrates 45.8g	**15%**
Dietary Fiber 3.6g	**15%**
Sugars 20.2g	
Protein 5.2g	

Vitamin A 62%	•	Vitamin C 3%
Calcium 10%	•	Iron 13%

Nutrition Grade C+

* Based on a 2000 calorie diet

Ingredients

- 1 large egg (separated)
- 1 teaspoon natural unsweetened applesauce
- 1 teaspoon canola oil
- 1/2 cup Z-Sweet stevia or Splenda (or unrefined brown sugar)
- 2 Tablespoon non-fat yogurt
- 1/2 teaspoon pure vanilla extract
- 1 cup gluten-free all-purpose white flour
- 1/2 cup gluten-free flour
- 1/4 teaspoon salt
- 1 teaspoon baking powder
- 1/4 teaspoon baking soda
- 3/4 teaspoon pumpkin pie spice
- 1 cup carrots (peeled and shredded)
- 1/4 cup quick-cooking oatmeal
- 1/2 cup low-fat buttermilk
- ½ cup chopped walnuts (optional)

Directions

1. Preheat oven to 375°F. Line a muffin tin with muffin papers. (Use a Texas sized muffin tin to get a half a dozen huge muffins.)
2. Separate egg yolk from the egg white, and then set the egg yolk aside. In a large bowl, whisk the egg white until foamy, and then add the canola oil and applesauce and whisk together until smooth. Mix in the Z-Sweet or Splenda, egg yolk, yogurt and vanilla extract, whisk until smooth.
3. Place the all-purpose flour, whole wheat flour, salt, baking powder, baking soda, pumpkin pie spice, and oatmeal in a sifter and sift into the mixing bowl.
4. Stir egg mixture into the flour and oatmeal mixture, just until moistened. Slowly fold the shredded carrots and walnuts into the mixture. Stir in the buttermilk until smooth.
5. Scoop batter into prepared muffin cups. Bake for 12 – 15 minutes, until a toothpick inserted into center of a muffin comes out clean.
6. Note: Muffins can be kept frozen in a tightly sealed plastic bag for 24-36 hours. Reheat gently.

7. Full-packed Granola

Servings: 6
Serving size: 1 medium-size bowl
Total time: 1 hour

Nutrition Facts

Serving Size 563 g

Amount Per Serving

Calories 267   Calories from Fat 85

     % Daily Value*

Total Fat 9.4g	**15%**
Saturated Fat 0.9g	**5%**
Trans Fat 0.0g	
Cholesterol 0mg	**0%**
Sodium 70mg	**3%**
Total Carbohydrates 37.4g	**12%**
Dietary Fiber 7.2g	**29%**
Sugars 10.2g	
Protein 9.1g	

Vitamin A 0% •	Vitamin C 2%
Calcium 7% •	Iron 14%

Nutrition Grade A-

* Based on a 2000 calorie diet

Ingredients

- 3 quarts water
- 1 1/3 cups steel cut oats
- 2/3 cup quinoa
- ¼ cup flaxseed/flax meal
- 1/4 cup sliced almonds
- 1/4 cup chopped walnuts
- 1/2 cup unsweetened applesauce
- 1/2 teaspoon ground cinnamon
- 1/2 teaspoon ground nutmeg
- 1/8 teaspoon salt
- 2 Tablespoon pure maple syrup
- 1/4 cup raisins
- 1/4 cup dried cranberries

Directions

1. Preheat oven to 300°F. Line two large baking sheets with parchment or aluminum foil.

2. In a large bowl, combine the oats, quinoa, almonds, and walnuts.
3. In a saucepan, stir together the salt, maple syrup, applesauce, cinnamon, and nutmeg. Bring to a boil over medium heat, then pour over the dry ingredients, and stir to coat. Spread the mixture out evenly on prepared baking sheets.
4. Bake in preheated oven for 45 minutes. Stir with a fork once halfway through. Let cool, and then stir in the raisins, cranberries, and flaxseeds. Store in an airtight container.

8. 15-minute Flax and Banana Oatmeal
Servings: 2
Serving size: 1 medium-size bowl
Total time: 15 minutes

Nutrition Facts

Serving Size 122 g

Amount Per Serving

Calories 139	Calories from Fat 13
	% Daily Value*
Total Fat 1.5g	**2%**
Trans Fat 0.0g	
Cholesterol 3mg	**1%**
Sodium 103mg	**4%**
Total Carbohydrates 25.3g	**8%**
Dietary Fiber 2.8g	**11%**
Sugars 15.8g	
Protein 6.9g	

Vitamin A 6%	•	Vitamin C 8%
Calcium 20%	•	Iron 4%

Nutrition Grade A

* Based on a 2000 calorie diet

Ingredients
- 1/2 cup quick cooking oats
- 2 tablespoons unrefined brown sugar (or honey)
- 1 1/2 cups fat free evaporated milk
- 1/4 teaspoon ground cinnamon
- 1 pinch salt
- 1 pinch ground nutmeg
- 2 large sliced bananas
- 2 tablespoon ground flaxseed

Directions

1. Stir together oats, sugar, milk, cinnamon, nutmeg, and salt in a saucepan.
2. Bring to a boil, stirring constantly for 2 minutes over low heat.
3. Add flaxseed and top with sliced bananas.

9. Fruit Polenta with Sesame seeds

Servings: 6
Serving size: 1 cup
Total time: 50 minutes

Nutrition Facts

Serving Size 186 g

Amount Per Serving

Calories 267   Calories from Fat 31

% Daily Value*

Total Fat 3.4g	**5%**
Saturated Fat 1.8g	**9%**
Trans Fat 0.0g	
Cholesterol 11mg	**4%**
Sodium 59mg	**2%**
Total Carbohydrates 54.4g	**18%**
Dietary Fiber 1.8g	**7%**
Sugars 20.2g	
Protein 3.1g	

Vitamin A 5%   •   Vitamin C 2%
Calcium 17%   •   Iron 5%

Nutrition Grade C

* Based on a 2000 calorie diet

Ingredients

- 1 cup instant polenta
- 3 cups low-fat (2%) milk
- 2 tablespoons unrefined brown sugar (or honey)
- Salt to taste
- 4 to 6 tablespoons blackberry jam
- 1 tablespoons Sesame seeds
- Lightly sweetened whipped crème fraîche (or use lightly sweetened dairy free sour cream)
- 1/4 cup raisins or 1/4 cup dried cranberries

Directions

1. Add 3 cups water and milk to a medium size saucepan and bring to a boil over medium heat. Turn the heat to low so liquid is barely boiling. Add the polenta and stir frequently to prevent lumps. Stir in sugar and salt.
2. Simmer and stir often for 20 to 40 minutes, until polenta is soft and creamy. Stir in the dried fruit.
3. Ladle polenta into bowls and top each serving with about 1 tablespoon blackberry jam and a spoonful of crème fraîche.

10. Chicken Tortilla Soup with Black Beans

Servings: 4
Serving size: 2 cups
Total time: 60 Minutes

Nutrition Facts

Serving Size 561 g

Amount Per Serving

Calories 456	Calories from Fat 109

	% Daily Value*
Total Fat 12.2g	**19%**
Saturated Fat 2.9g	**14%**
Trans Fat 0.0g	
Cholesterol 101mg	**34%**
Sodium 535mg	**22%**
Total Carbohydrates 47.0g	**16%**
Dietary Fiber 7.6g	**31%**
Sugars 5.7g	
Protein 40.9g	

Vitamin A 133%	•	Vitamin C 18%
Calcium 10%	•	Iron 28%

Nutrition Grade A-
* Based on a 2000 calorie diet

Ingredients

- 1 teaspoon extra virgin olive oil
- 1 large onion (diced)
- 2 ribs celery (diced)
- 2 large carrots (diced)
- 1 can (15 ounces) black beans, rinsed and drained
- 3 ears corn (cut kernels off cob)
- 1 lb boneless skinless chicken thighs (cubed)
- 2 teaspoon ground cumin

78

- 1 teaspoon Paprika
- 1 teaspoon chili powder
- 4 cups low-sodium chicken broth
- 1/2 teaspoon Salt
- Fresh ground black pepper (to taste)
- 16 tortilla chips
- ¼ cup fresh cilantro

Directions

1. In a medium stock pot, heat olive oil over medium high heat, cook and stir in the onion for 3 minutes.
2. Add the celery, black beans and carrots and cook for another 3 minutes, stirring frequently. Then add the broth, corn and chicken and cook for about 2 minutes. Add the cumin, paprika, chili powder, salt and pepper. Stir well.
3. Reduce heat to low and simmer for about 45 minutes, stirring occasionally.
4. Serve hot topped with crumbled tortilla chips and fresh cilantro.

11. Gluten-Free Chicken Noodle Soup

Servings: 6
Serving size: 1 cup
Total time: 30 minutes

Nutrition Facts

Serving Size 408 g

Amount Per Serving

Calories 196	Calories from Fat 40

% Daily Value*

Total Fat 4.4g	**7%**
Saturated Fat 0.5g	**3%**
Trans Fat 0.0g	
Cholesterol 32mg	**11%**
Sodium 458mg	**19%**
Total Carbohydrates 20.0g	**7%**
Dietary Fiber 1.7g	**7%**
Sugars 2.1g	
Protein 18.6g	

Vitamin A 62%	•	Vitamin C 4%
Calcium 3%	•	Iron 11%

Nutrition Grade A-

* Based on a 2000 calorie diet

Ingredients

- 1 tablespoon extra-virgin olive oil
- 1/2 cup chopped onion
- 1/2 cup chopped celery
- 6 cups low sodium chicken broth
- 1 (14.5 ounce) can vegetable broth
- 1/2 pound chopped cooked chicken breast
- 1 1/2 cups gluten-free egg noodles (or gluten-free fusilli, rotini or orzo)
- 1 cup sliced carrots
- 1/2 teaspoon dried basil
- 1/2 teaspoon dried oregano
- Salt and pepper to taste

Directions

1. Cook the egg noodles according to package directions in a medium pot. Set aside.
2. In a separate large pot over medium heat, sauté onion, celery, and carrots in olive oil for 5 minutes, or until tender.

3. Add the chicken, vegetable and chicken broths, basil, oregano, salt and pepper to the pot of veggies. Bring to a boil, reduce heat, cover and simmer for 20 minutes.
4. Add drained noodles to chicken and veggies, simmer for an additional 10 minutes.

12. Fruit 'N Oats Smoothie
Servings: 4
Total time: 5 minutes

Nutrition Facts

Serving Size 280 g

Amount Per Serving

Calories 232	Calories from Fat 33

	% Daily Value*
Total Fat 3.7g	**6%**
Saturated Fat 0.6g	**3%**
Trans Fat 0.0g	
Cholesterol 0mg	**0%**
Sodium 65mg	**3%**
Total Carbohydrates 42.6g	**14%**
Dietary Fiber 5.4g	**21%**
Sugars 18.3g	
Protein 7.8g	

Vitamin A 1%	•	Vitamin C 90%
Calcium 6%	•	Iron 11%

Nutrition Grade B+

* Based on a 2000 calorie diet

Ingredients
- 2 cup soy milk (or vitamin fortified soy milk/almond milk)
- 1 cup rolled oats
- 2 ripe bananas, sliced into chunks
- 25 frozen strawberries (or non-fat strawberry yogurt)
- 1 teaspoon vanilla extract
- 2 1/2 teaspoons unrefined brown sugar (or honey)

Directions
1. In a blender, puree the oats until it is powdery.
2. Add soy milk, oats, banana, strawberries, and sugar.
3. Blend until smooth. Pour into glasses and serve.

13. Spinach and Bacon Frittata

Servings: 3-4

Total time: 25 minutes

Nutrition Facts

Serving Size 300 g

Amount Per Serving	
Calories 269	Calories from Fat 183

	% Daily Value*
Total Fat 20.3g	**31%**
Saturated Fat 7.2g	**36%**
Trans Fat 0.0g	
Cholesterol 130mg	**43%**
Sodium 773mg	**32%**
Total Carbohydrates 5.8g	**2%**
Dietary Fiber 2.0g	**8%**
Sugars 1.4g	
Protein 13.9g	

Vitamin A 37%	•	Vitamin C 21%
Calcium 13%	•	Iron 8%

Nutrition Grade B-

* Based on a 2000 calorie diet

Ingredients

- 5/8 (10 ounce) package frozen chopped spinach, thawed and squeezed thoroughly to remove liquid
- 6 strips bacon, cut into bite-sized pieces
- 1 onion, chopped
- 1/2 cup Portobello mushrooms, chopped
- 3 eggs, beaten (or egg substitute)
- ¼ cup cheddar cheese, freshly grated (optional)
- 1 pinch dill or 1 pinch other herbs
- salt and pepper (to taste)
- 1 teaspoon extra-virgin olive oil

Directions

1. In a 10-inch nonstick broiler-proof skillet over medium heat, fry bacon until crispy. Drain the bacon and set aside. Remove the pan drippings.
2. Heat the extra-virgin olive oil and sauté the onions and mushrooms for 3 minutes. Add the spinach and cook until wilted. Return the bacon to the pan.

3. In a bowl, beat together the eggs, salt, and pepper. Slowly pour the egg mixture into the skillet, season with herbs, salt and pepper, to taste. Stir in the cheese. Cover and let cook for 2 minutes or until eggs start to set. Sprinkle cheese over the top.
4. Preheat broiler. Broil frittata for 3-5 minutes, or until center is set. Let cool, cut in wedges and serve.

LUNCH

14. Quick Mama Chicken Pot Pie
Servings: 6
Total time: 1 hour and 10 minutes

Nutrition Facts

Serving Size 238 g

Amount Per Serving

Calories 398　　　　Calories from Fat 155

	% Daily Value*
Total Fat 17.2g	**26%**
Saturated Fat 2.2g	**11%**
Trans Fat 0.0g	
Cholesterol 66mg	**22%**
Sodium 778mg	**32%**
Total Carbohydrates 30.4g	**10%**
Dietary Fiber 2.6g	**10%**
Sugars 6.5g	
Protein 29.5g	

Vitamin A 74%	•	Vitamin C 19%	
Calcium 9%	•	Iron 14%	

Nutrition Grade A-
* Based on a 2000 calorie diet

Ingredients
- 2 (9 inch) gluten free unbaked pie crusts (Kinnikinnick Gluten Free Pie Crusts)
- 1/2 cup Portobello mushrooms
- 1 cup frozen green peas
- 2 carrots, diced
- 1-1/2 pounds boneless, skinless chicken breast, cubed
- 3/4 teaspoon dried thyme

- 3/8 (10.75 ounce) can condensed cream of celery soup (or cream of chicken soup)
- 1 cup nonfat milk

Directions

1. Preheat oven to 400 degrees F (200 degrees C).
2. In a saucepan, combine chicken, mushrooms, carrots, peas. Add water to cover and boil for 15 minutes. Remove from heat, drain and set aside. In a separate saucepan over medium heat, cook thyme, celery soup and milk. Turn heat to medium-low, and simmer chicken mixture until thick. Remove from heat and set aside.
3. Unroll the pie crusts and gently fit 1 crust into a 9-inch pie pan. Place the chicken mixture in bottom pie crust. Pour the hot milk mixture over the chicken mixture. Lay second crust on top; seal edges and flute. Cut slits in several places on top crust to allow for steam to escape.
4. Bake for 30 minutes or until crust is golden brown. After 15 minutes of baking, cover crust edge with aluminum foil so they don't burn. Remove from oven and let stand for 5 minutes and then serve.

15. Cranberry Spinach Salad with Toasted Almonds
Servings: 5
Total time: 20 Minutes

Nutrition Facts

Serving Size 135 g

Amount Per Serving

Calories 226	Calories from Fat 162

% Daily Value*

Total Fat 18.0g	**28%**
Saturated Fat 2.2g	**11%**
Trans Fat 0.0g	
Cholesterol 0mg	**0%**
Sodium 62mg	**3%**
Total Carbohydrates 14.6g	**5%**
Dietary Fiber 3.8g	**15%**
Sugars 1.4g	
Protein 4.7g	

Vitamin A 128%	•	Vitamin C 35%
Calcium 13%	•	Iron 16%

Nutrition Grade B+

* Based on a 2000 calorie diet

Ingredients
- 2 teaspoons low-fat butter
- 1/2 cup and 1 tablespoon almonds, blanched and slivered
- 3/4 pound spinach, rinsed and torn into bite-size pieces
- 3/4 cup dried cranberries
- 2 tablespoons toasted sesame seeds
- 1/4 cup and 2 tablespoons unrefined brown sugar
- 1/8 teaspoon paprika
- 3 tablespoons white wine vinegar
- 3 tablespoons cider vinegar
- 1/4 cup and 2 tablespoons extra virgin olive oil

Directions
1. Melt butter in a saucepan over medium heat. Stir in almonds until lightly toasted. Remove from heat and let cool.
2. In a medium bowl, toss spinach with sesame seeds. Season with onion, paprika, sugar, white wine vinegar, cider vinegar, and vegetable oil. Add cranberries and toasted almonds.
3. Mix well and serve.

16. Wholesome Pasta Primavera
Servings: 6
Serving size: 2 cups
Total time: 30 minutes

Nutrition Facts
Serving Size 194 g

Amount Per Serving

Calories 221	Calories from Fat 93

	% Daily Value*
Total Fat 10.3g	**16%**
Saturated Fat 2.9g	**15%**
Trans Fat 0.0g	
Cholesterol 11mg	**4%**
Sodium 415mg	**17%**
Total Carbohydrates 25.3g	**8%**
Dietary Fiber 4.1g	**16%**
Sugars 4.5g	
Protein 8.1g	

Vitamin A 77%	•	Vitamin C 43%
Calcium 15%	•	Iron 12%

Nutrition Grade B
* Based on a 2000 calorie diet

Ingredients
- 1 cup carrots, sliced
- 1 cup fresh peas
- 1 cup mushrooms, sliced
- 1 cup snow peas or sugar snaps
- 1 cup asparagus spears, sliced
- 1 1/2 cloves garlic, chopped
- 1 lb. gluten-free penne
- 3 tablespoon extra-virgin olive oil
- ½ cup reduced-fat feta cheese, grated (optional)
- ½ cup shredded basil
- 1/3 teaspoon salt

Directions
1. Place vegetables in a steamer. Put the steamer in a large pot; add water (make sure base of steamer doesn't touch the water). Bring to a boil. Cover and steam for about 4 minutes or until tender. Rinse under cold running water and drain.

2. Boil water in a large pot. Add penne noodles and salt and cook uncovered until al dente. Drain the pasta and set aside.
3. Meanwhile, heat the olive oil in a large pan over low heat. Sauté garlic until lightly browned. Remove the garlic from the pan and discard it.
4. Add the steamed vegetables and turn the heat to medium. Cook for about 2-3 minutes. Add pasta and mix well. Sprinkle shredded basil and cheese on top and serve.

17. Pan Fried Cod with Cilantro Tartar Sauce

Servings: 4
Serving size: 4 ounces fish
Total time: 30 Minutes

Nutrition Facts

Serving Size 266 g

Amount Per Serving

Calories 318   Calories from Fat 127

	% Daily Value*
Total Fat 14.1g	**22%**
Saturated Fat 1.8g	**9%**
Trans Fat 0.0g	
Cholesterol 91mg	**30%**
Sodium 595mg	**25%**
Total Carbohydrates 15.2g	**5%**
Dietary Fiber 1.5g	**6%**
Sugars 2.6g	
Protein 34.1g	

Vitamin A 10%	•	Vitamin C 7%
Calcium 7%	•	Iron 11%

Nutrition Grade C
* Based on a 2000 calorie diet

Ingredients

Fried Cod:
- 2 large egg whites
- 4 Tablespoon coarse ground corn meal
- 1/4 teaspoon salt
- fresh ground black pepper (to taste)
- 4 (6-ounce) cod fillets (or other whitefish)
- 4 Tablespoon fresh dill
- 2 teaspoon extra-virgin olive oil

Cilantro Tartar Sauce:
- ½ cup low-fat mayonnaise
- 1 rib celery, diced
- ½ cup fresh cilantro leaves (coarsely chopped)
- 1 tablespoon fresh lime juice
- 1/8 teaspoon salt
- Fresh ground black pepper (to taste)

Directions

Cilantro Tartar Sauce:
Combine all ingredients and chill until ready to serve.

Pan Fried Cod:
1. Combine cornmeal, salt, and pepper in a bowl, stirring with a whisk. In a shallow dish, whisk egg whites until frothy.
2. Dredge each fish fillet in the egg white one at a time, and then sprinkle each side with dill. Dredge in the cornmeal mixture until well coated.
3. Heat olive oil in a large skillet over medium high heat. Add the coated fish and cook for about 6-7 minutes each side.
4. Serve topped with Cilantro tartar sauce.

18. Sautéed Veggies and Green Beans

Servings: 2
Serving size: 3 cups
Total time: 30 Minutes

Nutrition Facts

Serving Size 751 g

Amount Per Serving

Calories 389	Calories from Fat 191

% Daily Value*

Total Fat 21.3g	**33%**
Saturated Fat 6.5g	**33%**
Cholesterol 25mg	**8%**
Sodium 992mg	**41%**
Total Carbohydrates 44.6g	**15%**
Dietary Fiber 20.3g	**81%**
Sugars 12.3g	
Protein 15.8g	

Vitamin A 79%	•	Vitamin C 210%
Calcium 41%	•	Iron 42%

Nutrition Grade A

* Based on a 2000 calorie diet

Ingredients

- 2 tablespoon extra-virgin olive oil
- 1 cup yellow squash (diced)
- 1 medium zucchini (1/4 inch dice)
- 1 cup cauliflower, cut into small flowerets
- 3/4 cup celery, diced
- 2 pounds green beans stem end removed
- 1 Tablespoon dried oregano
- 1/2 teaspoon dried marjoram
- 1 teaspoon dried thyme
- 2 ounces feta cheese, crumbled (optional)
- 1/2 teaspoon salt
- fresh ground black pepper, to taste

Directions

1. Bring a large pot of water to a boil over medium heat. Add a pinch of salt and add the green beans. Cook for about 5 minutes. Drain and set aside.
2. In a large non-stick skillet, heat olive oil over medium-high heat. Add the cauliflower; sauté and toss occasionally until

golden brown. Stir in the celery and cook for about 3-5 minutes. Add squash, zucchini, oregano, marjoram and thyme, salt, and pepper.
3. Cook over medium-high heat for about 10 - 15 minutes tossing frequently. Add the blanched beans and let stand for a minute. Serve with crumbled feta cheese on top.

19. Two-Mushroom Risotto with Green Peas
Servings: 4
Total time: 35 minutes

Nutrition Facts
Serving Size 528 g

Amount Per Serving	
Calories 381	Calories from Fat 101

	% Daily Value*
Total Fat 11.2g	**17%**
Saturated Fat 3.2g	**16%**
Cholesterol 11mg	**4%**
Sodium 345mg	**14%**
Total Carbohydrates 50.8g	**17%**
Dietary Fiber 4.8g	**19%**
Sugars 3.9g	
Protein 16.9g	

Vitamin A 7%	Vitamin C 27%
Calcium 15%	Iron 24%

Nutrition Grade C+
* Based on a 2000 calorie diet

Ingredients
- 4 cups low sodium chicken broth, divided
- 2 tablespoons extra-virgin olive oil
- 11 ounces Portobello mushrooms, thinly sliced
- 11 ounces wild mushrooms, thinly sliced
- 1 small white onion, diced
- 1 cups Arborio rice
- 1/3 cup white wine (or white grape juice)
- 1/8 teaspoon salt
- freshly ground black pepper to taste
- 2 tablespoons fresh basil
- 3/4 cup green peas
- 1/2 cup freshly grated Parmesan cheese

Directions

1. Note: Soak onions in a cup of water for about 3 minutes before cooking. Drain.
2. In a medium sized stock-pot heat the olive oil over medium heat. Add diced onions and cook until translucent. Stir in the Portobello mushrooms and cook over medium-high heat until lightly brown, about 3 minutes. Continue to stir the mushrooms until they are dark roasted brown.
3. Add rice, stir frequently to coat with oil, about 2 minutes. Turn heat to medium and pour in wine. Stir well until the wine is fully absorbed, about 1 minute. Add 2 cups chicken broth to the rice and stir continuously until the liquid is absorbed and the rice is al dente, about 15 minutes. Add remaining broth, 1/4 cup at a time, allowing the rice to absorb each addition of broth before adding more.
4. When the rice is slightly firm and creamy but not mushy, stir in the basil, green peas, wild mushrooms and ¼ cup parmesan cheese. Stir and cook for another 2 - 3 minutes over very low heat. Season with salt and pepper to taste. Serve with freshly grated Parmesan.

20. Creamy Mushroom Soup
Servings: 6
Total time: 50 minutes

Nutrition Facts

Serving Size 143 g

Amount Per Serving

Calories 213   Calories from Fat 108

	% Daily Value*
Total Fat 12.1g	19%
Saturated Fat 4.0g	20%
Cholesterol 15mg	5%
Sodium 304mg	13%
Total Carbohydrates 15.1g	5%
Dietary Fiber 5.3g	21%
Sugars 0.6g	
Protein 7.6g	

Vitamin A 3%	•	Vitamin C 2%
Calcium 5%	•	Iron 20%

Nutrition Grade C+

* Based on a 2000 calorie diet

Ingredients

- 5 cups sliced fresh porcini mushrooms
- 1 1/2 cups chicken broth
- 1/2 cup chopped onion
- 1/8 teaspoon dried thyme
- 3 tablespoons extra-virgin olive oil
- 3 tablespoons gluten-free all-purpose flour
- 1/4 teaspoon salt
- 1/4 teaspoon ground black pepper
- 1 cup half-and-half
- 1 tablespoon sherry

Directions

1. In a heavy-based pan over medium heat, sauté the onions in 1 tablespoon olive oil until the onions were soft and clear. Add the mushrooms and cook on low heat for about 3 minutes. Add the thyme and cook for another 10- 15 minutes or until tender. Add 1/8 teaspoon salt.
2. Puree half of the mushroom mixture in a food processor or blender. Set aside.
3. Heat 2 tablespoon olive oil in the saucepan, whisk in flour until smooth. Add pepper, remaining salt, half and half and mushroom puree and mixture; stirring constantly. Bring soup to a boil and simmer until thickened. Season to taste, and pour in sherry.

21. Herbed Quinoa and Black Beans

Servings: 10

Total time: 50 minutes

Note: This recipe makes good leftovers.

Nutrition Facts

Serving Size 171 g

Amount Per Serving

Calories 226	Calories from Fat 25

% Daily Value*

Total Fat 2.8g	**4%**
Saturated Fat 0.8g	**4%**
Cholesterol 2mg	**1%**
Sodium 151mg	**6%**
Total Carbohydrates 39.1g	**13%**
Dietary Fiber 8.0g	**32%**
Sugars 2.1g	
Protein 12.7g	

Vitamin A 2%	•	Vitamin C 4%
Calcium 8%	•	Iron 17%

Nutrition Grade A

* Based on a 2000 calorie diet

Ingredients

- 1 teaspoon extra virgin olive oil
- 1 onion, chopped
- 2 cloves garlic, peeled and chopped
- 3/4 cup uncooked quinoa
- 1 (15 ounce) cans black beans, rinsed and drained
- 1 1/2 cups organic vegetable broth (or low-sodium chicken broth)
- 1/4 teaspoon cayenne pepper
- salt and pepper to taste
- 1 teaspoon ground cumin
- 1 cup frozen corn kernels
- 1/2 cup chopped fresh cilantro
- grated feta cheese (optional)
- 2 cups fresh water

Directions

1. Soak quinoa in fresh water for 15 minutes. Using a fine metal strainer or colander, rinse quinoa well before cooking.

2. In a medium saucepan, heat olive oil over medium heat. Add onion and garlic; sauté until beginning to soften, about 5 minutes.

3. Stir in quinoa, cayenne pepper, cumin, salt, and pepper and cover with vegetable broth. Bring the mixture to a boil over medium-high heat. Cover, reduce heat to medium-low, and simmer 20 minutes, or until broth is absorbed and quinoa is tender.

4. Add frozen corn, black beans, and ¼ cup cilantro, continue to simmer uncovered until heated through, about 5 minutes. Ladle into a bowl and sprinkle with ¼ cup cilantro and grated cheese.

22. Eggplant and Portobello Mushroom Omelet
Servings: 4
Total time: 35 minutes

Nutrition Facts

Serving Size 302 g

Amount Per Serving

Calories 260   Calories from Fat 152

	% Daily Value*
Total Fat 16.9g	**26%**
Saturated Fat 6.0g	**30%**
Cholesterol 104mg	**35%**
Sodium 431mg	**18%**
Total Carbohydrates 15.1g	**5%**
Dietary Fiber 8.1g	**32%**
Sugars 5.7g	
Protein 15.3g	

Vitamin A 7%	•	Vitamin C 15%
Calcium 29%	•	Iron 20%

Nutrition Grade A-

* Based on a 2000 calorie diet

Ingredients
- 4 medium sized Portobello mushrooms (stems removed and sliced)
- 2 medium sized Eggplant, peeled and diced
- 2 eggs
- ¼ teaspoon of black pepper
- 1/4 salt
- 2 tablespoon. extra virgin oil

- ½ cup of cilantro, finely chopped
- 1 cup shredded low-fat Parmesan cheese

Directions

1. Heat 1 tablespoon. olive oil in a medium skillet over medium heat. Add mushrooms and eggplant, sauté for 4-5 minutes until just tender. Add 1/8 teaspoon salt and 1/8 teaspoon pepper. Transfer to a bowl and set aside.
2. In a separate bowl, beat eggs with the milk and remaining salt and pepper.
3. Heat remaining olive oil (in the skillet used to cook the vegetables) over medium heat. Add the egg mixture and cook for 2 minutes. As the omelet begins to set, lift the edges to allow egg mixture to flow underneath.
4. Spoon quarter of the vegetable mixture into the center of the omelet, and sprinkle 1/4 cup of shredded parmesan cheese and cilantro on top of the omelet. Gently fold one edge of the omelet over the vegetables using a spatula. Cover and let cook for another 2 minutes or until cheese is melted. Transfer the omelet onto a plate and serve.

23. Hearty Garden Vegetable Soup

Servings: 4
Total time: 35 minutes

Nutrition Facts

Serving Size 261 g

Amount Per Serving

Calories 38   Calories from Fat 12

% Daily Value*

Total Fat 1.3g	**2%**
Trans Fat 0.0g	
Cholesterol 0mg	**0%**
Sodium 504mg	**21%**
Total Carbohydrates 5.4g	**2%**
Dietary Fiber 2.0g	**8%**
Sugars 2.4g	
Protein 1.8g	

Vitamin A 64%	•	Vitamin C 27%
Calcium 3%	•	Iron 2%

Nutrition Grade A

* Based on a 2000 calorie diet

Ingredients
- 1 teaspoon extra-virgin olive oil
- 2/3 cup sliced carrot
- 1/4 cup diced onion
- 3 cups fat free, low-sodium broth (beef, chicken or vegetable)
- 1 1/2 cups diced green cabbage
- 1/2 cup green beans
- 1/2 teaspoon dried basil
- 1/4 teaspoon dried oregano
- 1/4 teaspoon salt
- 1/2 cup diced zucchini

Directions
1. Heat olive oil in a large saucepan over low heat. Sauté the carrot and onion until softened, about 5 minutes.
2. Add broth, cabbage, green beans, and simmer, covered about 15 minutes or until beans are tender.
3. Add zucchini and simmer 3-4 minutes. Serve hot.

24. Herbed Sesame Chicken Kabobs
Servings: 4
Total Time: 10 minutes

Nutrition Facts

Serving Size 148 g

Amount Per Serving	
Calories 363	Calories from Fat 195

	% Daily Value*
Total Fat 21.6g	**33%**
Saturated Fat 4.2g	**21%**
Cholesterol 101mg	**34%**
Sodium 629mg	**26%**
Total Carbohydrates 8.7g	**3%**
Dietary Fiber 1.3g	**5%**
Sugars 5.4g	
Protein 34.8g	

Vitamin A 2%	•	Vitamin C 1%
Calcium 12%	•	Iron 16%

Nutrition Grade B-
* Based on a 2000 calorie diet

Ingredients
- 1 tablespoon sesame oil

- 1 1/2 tablespoons olive oil
- 3 tablespoons light soy sauce
- 2 tablespoons unrefined brown sugar
- 1/4 cup sesame seeds
- 1 pound boneless, skinless chicken breasts cut into 1-inch chunks
- 1/4 teaspoon ginger, chopped
- 2 teaspoons fresh rosemary, minced

Directions

1. Combine sesame oil, olive oil, soy sauce, ginger, brown sugar, rosemary, and sesame seeds in a bowl. Add the chicken to the mixture; turn to coat. Place in the fridge and marinate for at least 30 minutes and up to 2 hours.
2. Thread 3 chunks of chicken onto a skewer. Place kabobs on a baking sheet.
3. Bake at 350 degrees F for 8-10 minutes or until just cooked through and chicken juices run clear.

25. Tuna salad sandwich

Servings: 4
Total time: 15 minutes

Nutrition Facts

Serving Size 306 g

Amount Per Serving

Calories 401   Calories from Fat 125

	% Daily Value*
Total Fat 13.8g	**21%**
Saturated Fat 1.2g	**6%**
Trans Fat 0.0g	
Cholesterol 23mg	**8%**
Sodium 458mg	**19%**
Total Carbohydrates 66.9g	**22%**
Dietary Fiber 18.0g	**72%**
Sugars 7.9g	
Protein 19.7g	

Vitamin A 9%	•	Vitamin C 78%
Calcium 2%	•	Iron 39%

Nutrition Grade B

* Based on a 2000 calorie diet

Ingredients

- 1 (7 ounce) can low-sodium white tuna,
- 6 tablespoons low-fat mayonnaise or low-fat salad dressing
- 3 tablespoons low-sodium sweet pickle relish
- 1/8 teaspoon dried onion flakes, minced
- 1 tablespoon dried parsley
- 1 teaspoon dried dill weed
- 1 tablespoon cilantro, minced
- 3 tablespoons ginger, minced
- Salt and pepper to taste
- 6 small inner leaves, romaine lettuce, cut into fine shreds
- 8 gluten-free breads (some Gluten-Free brands: Udi's, Kinnikinnick Foods, Food for Life, Glutino)

Directions

1. Drain and flake tuna. In a medium bowl, combine the tuna, onion flakes, and sweet pickle relish.
2. For dressing, combine mayonnaise, ginger, dill, parsley, cilantro in a small bowl, season with salt and pepper to taste. Blend well.
3. Add dressing to tuna mixture; toss to coat. Cover and chill for 5 minutes before serving.
4. Just before serving, stir in the shreds of romaine lettuce. Fill the breads and serve.

26. Mustard Turkey Burgers

Servings: 4

Total time: 30 Minutes

Nutrition Facts

Serving Size 275 g

Amount Per Serving

Calories 583	Calories from Fat 235

	% Daily Value*
Total Fat 26.1g	**40%**
Saturated Fat 8.3g	**41%**
Trans Fat 0.0g	
Cholesterol 211mg	**70%**
Sodium 732mg	**30%**
Total Carbohydrates 44.8g	**15%**
Dietary Fiber 4.8g	**19%**
Sugars 6.4g	
Protein 43.2g	

Vitamin A 5%	•	Vitamin C 2%
Calcium 24%	•	Iron 24%

Nutrition Grade C+

* Based on a 2000 calorie diet

Ingredients

- 1 pound ground turkey (breast is better)
- 1/4 teaspoon salt
- 1/8 teaspoon fresh ground black pepper
- 1 tablespoon Dijon mustard
- 1 teaspoon extra virgin olive oil
- 1/4 teaspoon dried thyme leaves
- 1 large egg
- 2 3/4 ounce slices reduced fat Swiss cheese
- 1 Tablespoon non-fat mayonnaise (per serving)
- Lettuce
- 4 Cucumber slices
- 8 whole wheat or gluten-free hamburger buns

Directions

1. Place a non-stick grill pan in the oven. Preheat to 375°F.
2. In a large bowl, combine ground turkey, salt, pepper, olive oil, mustard and thyme leaves and egg. Form mixture into 4 patties.

3. Place the burgers in the grill pan. Cook on the first side for 10 minutes, and 5 - 7 minutes on the other side. Top with the cheese and cook until the cheese is melted.
4. Serve on buns with 1 tablespoon non-fat mayonnaise, lettuce and cucumber.

DINNER

27. Ginger Halibut 'N Vegetables

Servings: 4
Total time: 25 Minutes

Nutrition Facts

Serving Size 406 g

Amount Per Serving

Calories 256	Calories from Fat 75

	% Daily Value*
Total Fat 8.4g	**13%**
Saturated Fat 1.4g	**7%**
Cholesterol 113mg	**38%**
Sodium 615mg	**26%**
Total Carbohydrates 7.8g	**3%**
Dietary Fiber 2.5g	**10%**
Sugars 3.0g	
Protein 41.5g	

Vitamin A 9%	•	Vitamin C 137%
Calcium 3%	•	Iron 39%

Nutrition Grade B-

* Based on a 2000 calorie diet

Ingredients

- 4 8-ounce skinless halibut fillets, sliced into 1 inch thick (or blue-eyed cod)
- 3 yellow squash or zucchini, cut into 1/2-inch rounds
- 1 head broccoli, cut into bite-size florets
- 4 teaspoons grated fresh ginger
- 1/8 teaspoon black pepper
- 2 tablespoons finely fresh flat-leaf parsley, chopped
- 4 teaspoons extra-virgin olive oil
- 1/2 teaspoon salt

Directions

1. Place a steamer in a large saucepan of boiling water. (If steamer is not available, put a ceramic dish or metal colander into a large covered skillet with water).
2. Add the vegetables and cover. Steam for about 7 minutes or until tender. Transfer vegetables to a bowl and season with 1/4 teaspoon salt. Cover to keep warm.
3. Sprinkle the halibut with ginger and season with the remaining salt and the pepper. Place the halibut on the steamer, cover and steam for 7 minutes or until fish is cooked depending on its thickness.
4. Drizzle the halibut and vegetables with olive oil and serve with chopped parsley on top.

28. 10-minute Sautéed Scallops

Servings: 2

Total time: 10 minutes

Nutrition Facts

Serving Size 253 g

Amount Per Serving

Calories 363   Calories from Fat 153

	% Daily Value*
Total Fat 17.0g	**26%**
Saturated Fat 2.4g	**12%**
Cholesterol 75mg	**25%**
Sodium 440mg	**18%**
Total Carbohydrates 13.3g	**4%**
Dietary Fiber 1.6g	**6%**
Protein 38.6g	

Vitamin A 4%	•	Vitamin C 14%
Calcium 9%	•	Iron 9%

Nutrition Grade B

* Based on a 2000 calorie diet

Ingredients

- 2 tablespoon extra-virgin olive oil
- 1 pound sea scallops
- 2 sprigs fresh rosemary
- 1 Tablespoon low-fat unsalted butter
- fresh ground black pepper (to taste)
- 1/16 teaspoon salt

Directions

1. Heat olive oil in medium-size saucepan over medium-high heat.
2. Add the scallops and season with salt and pepper. Stir in rosemary.
3. Cook each side of the scallop for 4 minutes. Serve hot.

29. Italian Chicken Marsala

Servings: 4
Total time: 30 minutes

Nutrition Facts

Serving Size 111 g

Amount Per Serving

Calories 167 — Calories from Fat 70

	% Daily Value*
Total Fat 7.8g	**12%**
Saturated Fat 2.3g	**12%**
Trans Fat 0.0g	
Cholesterol 38mg	**13%**
Sodium 141mg	**6%**
Total Carbohydrates 6.3g	**2%**
Dietary Fiber 1.1g	**5%**
Protein 12.5g	

Vitamin A 2%	•	Vitamin C 1%
Calcium 2%	•	Iron 10%

Nutrition Grade C-

* Based on a 2000 calorie diet

Ingredients

- 4 boneless, skinless chicken breast halves
- 2 Tablespoons gluten-free all-purpose Flour
- 1 Tablespoon low-fat Butter
- 1 tablespoon extra-virgin olive oil
- 1 Cup fresh Mushrooms, sliced
- 1/2 Cup Marsala Wine
- 2 Tablespoons Fresh Parsley, Chopped
- 1/4 Teaspoon Rosemary
- 1/8 teaspoon ground black pepper

Directions

1. Mix the flour and pepper in a medium bowl. Dredge chicken in the mixture to lightly coat.

2. In a large skillet, heat olive oil and butter over medium heat. Fry the chicken in the skillet for 4 minutes each side. Add mushrooms and cook until brown, mix well.
3. Pour Marsala wine, parsley and rosemary over the chicken. Turn heat to low and cover skillet. Simmer for 10 minutes.

30. Spinach and Zucchini Lasagna

Servings: 4
Total time: 1 hour, 14 minutes

Nutrition Facts

Serving Size 423 g

Amount Per Serving

Calories 393	Calories from Fat 173

	% Daily Value*
Total Fat 19.2g	**30%**
Saturated Fat 5.6g	**28%**
Trans Fat 0.1g	
Cholesterol 22mg	**7%**
Sodium 969mg	**40%**
Total Carbohydrates 25.6g	**9%**
Dietary Fiber 4.0g	**16%**
Sugars 4.4g	
Protein 31.4g	

Vitamin A 176%	•	Vitamin C 71%
Calcium 35%	•	Iron 21%

Nutrition Grade B+

* Based on a 2000 calorie diet

Ingredients

- 2 1/2 cups zucchini, cubed
- 12 oz gluten-free fresh lasagna noodles
- 12 oz. spinach leaves
- 2 teaspoon extra-virgin olive oil
- 1 1/2 cups low-fat carbonara sauce
- 2 cloves garlic, minced
- 1/2 teaspoon dried basil
- 1/8 teaspoon freshly ground pepper
- 1/2 teaspoon Kosher salt
- 2 cups low-fat cottage cheese (or low fat/ fat free ricotta)
- 2 1/2 cups low-fat mozzarella cheese, grated
- 1/4 cup low-fat parmesan cheese, grated

Directions

1. Preheat oven to 350 F.
2. Boil pasta until al dente (refer to package instructions). Strain and set aside.
3. Sprinkle cubed zucchini with salt and pepper. Place on a baking sheet and roast in the oven, about 15-20 minutes.
4. In a large pan over medium heat, sauté garlic in olive oil for 2-3 minutes or until fragrant. Stir in spinach and cook until the moisture is removed.
5. Transfer cooked spinach into a large bowl and mix in cottage cheese with some pepper to taste. Add salt if needed.
6. In a 9x13-inch casserole dish, spread a layer of carbonara sauce on bottom of the dish; arrange half of the noodles over the carbonara sauce; spread half of the cooked spinach on top; put all of the zucchini; top with half of the mozzarella; spread a layer of carbonara sauce; add the rest of the noodles; spread the rest of the cooked spinach; add the rest of the mozzarella; spread the rest of the carbonara sauce and top with all of the parmesan.
7. Bake for 40-45 minutes until bubbling and brown. Allow to cool slightly and serve.

31. Stir-Fried Ginger Shrimp 'N Vegetables

Servings: 4

Total time: 15 minutes

Nutrition Facts

Serving Size 287 g

Amount Per Serving

Calories 265	Calories from Fat 112

% Daily Value*

Total Fat 12.4g	**19%**
Saturated Fat 1.9g	**9%**
Trans Fat 0.0g	
Cholesterol 223mg	**74%**
Sodium 468mg	**19%**
Total Carbohydrates 11.7g	**4%**
Dietary Fiber 2.3g	**9%**
Sugars 2.0g	
Protein 28.5g	

Vitamin A 3%	•	Vitamin C 189%
Calcium 5%	•	Iron 32%

Nutrition Grade B-

* Based on a 2000 calorie diet

Ingredients

- 3 tablespoon extra-virgin olive oil and deveined
- 1lb. raw medium shrimp, peeled
- 2 cups broccoli florets
- 2 cups sliced mushrooms
- 4 scallions, trimmed and chopped
- 1 tablespoon Garlic, minced
- 2 tablespoon fresh ginger, minced
- 1 cup vegetable broth, mixed with 2 tablespoon cornstarch
- Salt and pepper to taste

Directions

1. In a wok or large skillet, heat olive oil over high heat until just smoking. Stir in garlic, scallions, and ginger. Cook until garlic just begins to brown.
2. Stir in broccoli and mushrooms, and continue cooking until tender, about 3 minutes.
3. Add shrimp, cook and continue to stir until they turn pink, about 3 minutes. Add vegetable broth and cover for 1

minute, stir until thickened. Season with salt and pepper, and serve.

32. Roast Pork 'N Herbs

Servings: 4
Total time: 50 minutes

Nutrition Facts

Serving Size 117 g

Amount Per Serving

Calories 170	Calories from Fat 39

% Daily Value*

Total Fat 4.4g	**7%**
Saturated Fat 1.5g	**8%**
Trans Fat 0.0g	
Cholesterol 83mg	**28%**
Sodium 66mg	**3%**
Total Carbohydrates 1.3g	**0%**
Dietary Fiber 0.8g	**3%**
Protein 29.9g	

Vitamin A 3%	•	Vitamin C 4%
Calcium 4%	•	Iron 14%

Nutrition Grade A
* Based on a 2000 calorie diet

Ingredients
- 1 pound pork tenderloin
- 1 tablespoon finely chopped rosemary
- 1 tablespoon finely chopped thyme
- 1 tablespoon finely chopped sage
- 1 tablespoon finely chopped parsley
- Salt and pepper to taste
- Extra-virgin olive oil spray

Directions
1. Spray pork lightly with extra-virgin olive oil. Combine thyme, sage, rosemary, parsley, salt, and pepper in small bowl. Rub mixture into the pork tenderloin. Cover and refrigerate for 6-8 hours, or overnight.
2. Preheat oven to 450 degrees F. Trim excess fat from pork.
3. Place the pork tenderloin in a shallow roasting pan, and roast for 30-35 minutes or until the internal temperature of the roast is 165 degrees F and the juices run clear.

4. Slice the pork tenderloin and serve.

33. Mac 'N Tuna Casserole
Servings: 6
Total time: 55 minutes

Nutrition Facts

Serving Size 92 g

Amount Per Serving	
Calories 176	Calories from Fat 12
	% Daily Value*
Total Fat 1.3g	**2%**
Trans Fat 0.0g	
Cholesterol 5mg	**2%**
Sodium 29mg	**1%**
Total Carbohydrates 31.8g	**11%**
Dietary Fiber 4.9g	**20%**
Sugars 2.4g	
Protein 8.9g	
Vitamin A 7% •	Vitamin C 17%
Calcium 1% •	Iron 9%

Nutrition Grade B
* Based on a 2000 calorie diet

Ingredients
- 8 oz gluten-free elbow macaroni (or wide egg noodles), uncooked
- 1 can (6 oz) water-packed tuna, drained, flaked in bite-size pieces
- 1 cup frozen green peas, thawed
- 1 cup sliced celery
- 1 can (10 3/4 oz) reduced-fat cream of celery soup, undiluted (or 2 cans Campbell's Healthy Request Cream of Mushroom Soup)
- 1 tablespoon chopped fresh rosemary or 1 teaspoon dried
- 1/2 cup skim or 1% milk
- 1 cup shredded, reduced-fat sharp cheddar cheese
- 1/2 cup low-fat mayonnaise
- 2 ounces Parmigiano-Reggiano (grated)
- Spray olive oil

Directions

1. Cook macaroni in a large pot of boiling salted water until tender. Drain. Rinse under cold water and drain again. Combine cooked macaroni, tuna, green peas, rosemary, and celery in a mixing bowl. Set aside.
2. In a small saucepan, simmer soup and milk over medium heat until smooth. Add cheese and continue to heat until cheese is melted. Remove soup from heat. Stir in mayonnaise to soup until well blended. Pour soup over macaroni mixture. Fold together gently.
3. Spray a 1 ½ quart casserole dish with non-stick spray. Pour macaroni and soup mixture into casserole dish, and sprinkle the cheese over the top.
4. Bake at 350 degrees, uncovered for 30 minutes.

34. Ginger Veggie and Tofu Stir-Fry

Servings: 6
Total time: 40 minutes

Nutrition Facts

Serving Size 156 g

Amount Per Serving	
Calories 138	Calories from Fat 98

	% Daily Value*
Total Fat 10.9g	**17%**
Saturated Fat 1.6g	**8%**
Trans Fat 0.0g	
Cholesterol 0mg	**0%**
Sodium 958mg	**40%**
Total Carbohydrates 6.2g	**2%**
Dietary Fiber 1.4g	**6%**
Sugars 1.9g	
Protein 5.8g	

Vitamin A 4%	•	Vitamin C 73%
Calcium 9%	•	Iron 8%

Nutrition Grade B

* Based on a 2000 calorie diet

Ingredients

- 1 tablespoon cornstarch
- 1 1/2 cloves garlic, crushed
- 2 teaspoons chopped fresh ginger root, divided
- 1/4 cup extra-virgin olive oil, divided

- 1 14-ounce package soft tofu, drained and cut into 1-inch cubes
- 1 small head broccoli, cut into florets
- 1/2 cup snow peas
- 3/4 cup julienned carrots
- 1/2 cup halved green beans
- 2 tablespoons soy sauce
- 2 1/2 tablespoons water
- 1/4 cup chopped onion
- 1/2 tablespoon salt

Directions

1. Whisk soy sauce, cornstarch and water in a small bowl. Set aside.
2. Heat olive oil in a large skillet over medium heat. Sauté 1 teaspoon ginger and garlic until garlic is lightly brown. Add vegetables and tofu and cook for 2 minutes, stirring constantly to prevent burning. Pour soy sauce-cornstarch mixture into skillet.
3. Mix in onion, salt, and remaining 1 teaspoon ginger. Cook until vegetables are tender but still crisp. Serve over rice.

35. Herb and Chicken Soup

Servings: 6

Total time: 1hour and 40 minutes

Nutrition Facts

Serving Size 575 g

Amount Per Serving

Calories 443   Calories from Fat 268

% **Daily Value***

Total Fat 29.8g	**46%**
Saturated Fat 9.5g	**47%**
Trans Fat 0.0g	
Cholesterol 203mg	**68%**
Sodium 944mg	**39%**
Total Carbohydrates 2.3g	**1%**
Dietary Fiber 0.7g	**3%**
Sugars 1.4g	
Protein 40.9g	

Vitamin A 12%	•	Vitamin C 16%
Calcium 2%	•	Iron 2%

Nutrition Grade D

* Based on a 2000 calorie diet

Ingredients

- 5/8 (3 pound) whole rotisserie chicken, cut into quarters
- 2-1/2 medium sized carrots, diced
- 2-1/2 stalks celery, diced
- 1 medium sized onion, diced
- ½ cup parsley, chopped
- 1 bay leaf
- 2-1/2 quarts cold water
- salt and pepper to taste

Directions

1. Place chicken in a large pot and cover with water. Add 2 teaspoons salt and bay leaf. Cover the pot and bring to a boil. Uncover and skim off top foam.
2. Simmer, uncovered, about 1 hour (skim off fat).
3. Add onions, carrots, celery, and parsley and simmer for 30 minutes.

36. Rosemary Poached Chicken
Servings: 3-4
Total time: 50 minutes

Nutrition Facts

Serving Size 244 g

Amount Per Serving	
Calories 233	Calories from Fat 77
	% Daily Value*
Total Fat 8.5g	**13%**
Saturated Fat 2.3g	**12%**
Trans Fat 0.0g	
Cholesterol 101mg	**34%**
Sodium 441mg	**18%**
Total Carbohydrates 3.4g	**1%**
Dietary Fiber 1.1g	**4%**
Sugars 1.6g	
Protein 33.6g	

Vitamin A 105%	•	Vitamin C 4%	
Calcium 3%	•	Iron 9%	

Nutrition Grade B

* Based on a 2000 calorie diet

Ingredients
- 2 boneless skinless chicken breasts (about 1 pound)
- 1 1/2 – 2 cups fat free, low sodium chicken broth, or water
- 2 carrots, peeled and coarsely chopped
- 2 stalks celery, coarsely chopped
- 1 bay leaf
- 2 sprigs rosemary
- ¼ teaspoon salt

Directions
1. Place carrots, celery, bay leaf, rosemary and salt in a large pot, cover with broth or water and bring to a boil over high heat.
2. Add the chicken and bring back to a boil. Reduce heat to low and simmer for 10 minutes, or until cooked through. Let chicken sit in the warm liquid for 15-20 minutes.
3. Remove chicken from the broth, slice or shred and serve.

37. Rosemary Turkey and Quinoa Meatloaf

Servings: 5

Total time: 1 Hour 20 Minutes

Nutrition Facts

Serving Size 224 g

Amount Per Serving

Calories 362	Calories from Fat 156

	% Daily Value*
Total Fat 17.3g	**27%**
Saturated Fat 4.3g	**22%**
Trans Fat 0.0g	
Cholesterol 148mg	**49%**
Sodium 416mg	**17%**
Total Carbohydrates 16.9g	**6%**
Dietary Fiber 1.2g	**5%**
Sugars 10.0g	
Protein 33.5g	

Vitamin A 1%	•	Vitamin C 3%
Calcium 5%	•	Iron 17%

Nutrition Grade B+

* Based on a 2000 calorie diet

Ingredients

- 1/4 cup quinoa
- 1/2 cup water
- 1 teaspoon extra-virgin olive oil
- 1 small onion, chopped
- 1 clove garlic, chopped
- 1 (20 ounce) package ground turkey
- 2 tablespoons low-sodium gluten-free Worcestershire sauce (Lea & Perrins Worcestershire sauce)
- 1 egg, beaten
- 1/2 teaspoons salt
- 1 teaspoon freshly ground black pepper
- 2-3/4 teaspoons chopped fresh rosemary
- 1/3 cup and 2 tablespoons unrefined brown sugar
- 1 teaspoon water

Directions

1. In a saucepan, bring quinoa and water to a boil over high heat. Turn heat to medium-low, cover and simmer quinoa

for 15-20 minutes or until tender and water has been absorbed. Let cool and set aside.

2. Preheat an oven to 350 degrees F (175 degrees C).

3. Sauté onions in olive oil in a skillet over medium heat. Stir until softened and translucent, about 5 minutes. Add garlic and sauté for 1 minute. Remove from heat and let cool.

4. In a large bowl, combine turkey, cooked quinoa, onions, 2 tablespoons Worcestershire, egg, rosemary, salt, and pepper. Shape into a loaf on a foil lined baking sheet. Blend together brown sugar, 2 teaspoons Worcestershire, and 1 teaspoon water in a small bowl. Pour and rub evenly over the top of the loaf.

5. Bake for 50 minutes in the oven, or until no longer pink in the center. A thermometer inserted into the center should read at least 160 degrees F. Let meatloaf cool for 10 minutes, slice and serve.

38. Chicken 'N Spinach Feta Pasta

Servings: 4
Total time: 40 minutes

Nutrition Facts

Serving Size 282 g

Amount Per Serving		
Calories 560	Calories from Fat 208	
		% Daily Value*
Total Fat 23.1g		**35%**
Saturated Fat 9.9g		**49%**
Trans Fat 0.0g		
Cholesterol 117mg		**39%**
Sodium 962mg		**40%**
Total Carbohydrates 52.1g		**17%**
Dietary Fiber 1.6g		**6%**
Sugars 4.8g		
Protein 36.8g		
Vitamin A 47%	•	Vitamin C 14%
Calcium 32%	•	Iron 14%

Nutrition Grade B
* Based on a 2000 calorie diet

Ingredients

- 1 (8 ounce) package gluten-free penne pasta
- 2-1/2 cups cubed cooked chicken breast

113

- 2 tablespoons extra-virgin olive oil
- 1/2 cup chopped onion
- 1 clove garlic, minced
- ½ cup reduced fat milk (2%, 1% or skim)
- 1 cup sliced fresh mushrooms
- 3 cups spinach leaves, packed
- salt and pepper to taste
- 8 ounces feta cheese, crumbled

Directions
1. Boil pasta in a large pot of lightly salted water until al dente. Drain and set aside.
2. In a large skillet over medium-high heat, sauté onion and garlic in olive oil until golden brown.
3. Add mushrooms, chicken, and spinach. Season with salt and pepper. Cook until spinach is wilted, about 2 minutes.
4. Reduce heat to medium, stir in pasta, milk and feta cheese, and cook until heated through.

39. Zesty Baked Salmon
Servings: 2
Serving size: 1 fillet
Total time: 35 minutes

Nutrition Facts

Serving Size 213 g

Amount Per Serving

Calories 373   Calories from Fat 190

	% Daily Value*
Total Fat 21.1g	**33%**
Saturated Fat 4.3g	**22%**
Trans Fat 0.0g	
Cholesterol 107mg	**36%**
Sodium 2053mg	**86%**
Total Carbohydrates 3.6g	**1%**
Dietary Fiber 0.8g	**3%**
Sugars 0.7g	
Protein 39.9g	

Vitamin A 14%	•	Vitamin C 29%
Calcium 5%	•	Iron 10%

Nutrition Grade B+

* Based on a 2000 calorie diet

Ingredients

- 12 ounces salmon fillets (about 2 fillets)
- 1/4 cup soy sauce
- 1 teaspoon lemon juice
- 1/2 teaspoon ginger
- 1/4 teaspoon cinnamon
- 1/4 cup fresh parsley, Chopped
- 1/8 teaspoon pepper, freshly ground
- 1/8 teaspoon salt, freshly ground

Directions

1. Preheat oven to 325 degrees.
2. Wash salmon and pat dry. Place salmon in a shallow baking dish. Set aside.
3. In a bowl, mix together soy sauce, lemon juice, parsley, cinnamon, and ginger. Season with salt and pepper. Pour liquid mixture over the filets.
4. Bake for about 25 minutes or until salmon is flaky.

DESSERTS

40. Carrot Cake with Walnuts
Servings: 15 (makes 8x12 inch pan)
Total time: 1 Hour 40 Minutes
Note: This recipe makes good leftovers.

Nutrition Facts

Serving Size 100 g

Amount Per Serving

Calories 287 Calories from Fat 100

% **Daily Value***

Total Fat 11.1g **17%**

Saturated Fat 2.7g **14%**

Trans Fat 0.0g

Cholesterol 33mg **11%**

Sodium 247mg **10%**

Total Carbohydrates 43.0g **14%**

Dietary Fiber 2.0g **8%**

Sugars 21.7g

Protein 5.6g

Vitamin A 50% • Vitamin C 3%

Calcium 5% • Iron 10%

Nutrition Grade C-

* Based on a 2000 calorie diet

<="" p="">

Ingredients

- 3/4 cup low-fat buttermilk
- 1/4 cup extra-virgin olive oil
- 2 cups gluten-free all-purpose flour
- 2 cups carrots, shredded
- 2 teaspoons baking soda
- 3 eggs, beaten
- 1 cup flaked coconut
- 1 cup walnuts, chopped
- 1 cup raisins
- 1 1/2 cups unrefined brown sugar
- 2 teaspoons ground cinnamon
- 2 teaspoons vanilla extract
- 1/4 teaspoon salt

Directions

1. Preheat oven to 350 degrees F (175 degrees C). Grease and flour an 8x12 inch pan.
2. Sift together baking soda, flour, salt and cinnamon in a medium bowl. Set aside.
3. In a large bowl, combine buttermilk, eggs, oil, vanilla, and sugar. Mix in flour mixture. In a medium bowl, combine coconut, carrots, raisins and walnuts. Add carrot mixture to

batter and fold in well using a heavy whisk. Pour into prepared 8x12 inch pan.

4. Bake for 1 hour. Check with a toothpick by inserting it into center of a cake. The cake is cooked if the toothpick comes out clean or with only a few crumbs sticking to it. Let cool for at least 20 minutes before serving.

41. Gingery Fruit Salad

Servings: 4

Total time: 20 Minutes

Nutrition Facts

Serving Size 193 g

Amount Per Serving

Calories 202	Calories from Fat 90

% Daily Value*

Total Fat 10.0g	**15%**
Saturated Fat 1.1g	**6%**
Trans Fat 0.0g	
Cholesterol 3mg	**1%**
Sodium 42mg	**2%**
Total Carbohydrates 22.6g	**8%**
Dietary Fiber 4.0g	**16%**
Sugars 16.1g	
Protein 7.2g	

Vitamin A 2%	•	Vitamin C 12%
Calcium 12%	•	Iron 4%

Nutrition Grade B+

* Based on a 2000 calorie diet

Ingredients

- 1 red apple, cored and chopped
- 1 green apple, cored and chopped
- 1/2 cup green grapes
- 1/2 cup dried cranberries
- 1/4 cup finely chopped crystallized ginger (1 1/2 oz)
- 1/2 cup chopped walnuts
- 1 (8 ounce) container nonfat plain yogurt (or nonfat strawberry yogurt)

Directions

Note: It's best to put in the dried cranberries and walnuts right before serving to keep cranberries firm and walnuts crunchy.

1. In a large bowl, combine the first six ingredients.
2. Strain the yogurt with double cheesecloth or coffee filter.
3. Pour in yogurt and blend well. Chill until ready to serve.

42. Banana Cinnamon Crumb Muffins
Servings: 6
Total time: 35 Minutes

Nutrition Facts

Serving Size 65 g

Amount Per Serving

Calories 174   Calories from Fat 41

	% Daily Value*
Total Fat 4.5g	**7%**
Saturated Fat 2.7g	**13%**
Trans Fat 0.0g	
Cholesterol 17mg	**6%**
Sodium 250mg	**10%**
Total Carbohydrates 30.0g	**10%**
Dietary Fiber 0.6g	**2%**
Sugars 10.3g	
Protein 3.0g	

Vitamin A 1%	•	Vitamin C 3%
Calcium 3%	•	Iron 3%

Nutrition Grade F
* Based on a 2000 calorie diet

Ingredients
- 3/4 cup and 2 ½ tablespoons gluten-free all-purpose flour
- 1/2 teaspoon baking soda
- 1/2 teaspoon baking powder
- 1-3/4 bananas, mashed
- 1/3 cup and 5 1/4 tablespoons unrefined brown sugar
- 1/4 teaspoon salt
- 5/8 egg
- 1 tablespoon and 1/2 teaspoon gluten-free all-purpose flour
- 3 tablespoons and 1/2 teaspoon low-fat butter, melted
- 1/8 teaspoon ground cinnamon
- 1/2 teaspoon vanilla extract
- 1-3/4 teaspoons low-fat butter

Directions

1. Preheat oven to 375 degrees F (190 degrees C). Line 6 muffin cups with muffin papers.
2. Combine 3/4 cup and 2 ½ tablespoons flour, baking powder, baking soda, and salt in a large bowl. In another bowl, beat the sugar, melted butter and egg. Add the mashed banana and combine thoroughly; stirring just until moistened. Divide the batter among the prepared muffin cups.
3. In a small bowl, combine sugar, 1 tablespoon and 1/2 teaspoon flour, cinnamon, and vanilla. Mix in 1 tablespoon butter until the mixture becomes coarse. Sprinkle topping over muffins.
4. Bake for 18 to 20 minutes. Insert a toothpick into the center of each muffin; if it comes out clean it's done, else return the muffins to the oven and bake for a few more minutes.

43. Raisin Oatmeal Cookies

Servings: 6
Total time: 2 hours

Nutrition Facts

Serving Size 59 g

Amount Per Serving

Calories 184   Calories from Fat 41

	% Daily Value*
Total Fat 4.5g	**7%**
Saturated Fat 2.5g	**12%**
Trans Fat 0.0g	
Cholesterol 0mg	**0%**
Sodium 192mg	**8%**
Total Carbohydrates 34.4g	**11%**
Dietary Fiber 1.8g	**7%**
Sugars 19.0g	
Protein 2.7g	

Vitamin A 0%	•	Vitamin C 0%
Calcium 3%	•	Iron 9%

Nutrition Grade D+

* Based on a 2000 calorie diet

Ingredients

- 1/4 cup low-fat butter, softened
- 1/2 cup unrefined brown sugar

- 1/4 teaspoon vanilla extract
- 1/2 cup gluten-free all-purpose flour
- 1/4 teaspoon baking soda
- 1/8 cup boiling water
- 1/4 teaspoon salt
- 1/4 teaspoon ground cinnamon
- 3/4 cup quick cooking oats
- 1/2 cup raisins

Directions

1. Beat together butter, sugar, and egg in a bowl. Stir in vanilla until light and fluffy.
2. In another bowl, combine flour, salt, and cinnamon; put into the creamed mixture and stir well. Dissolve baking soda in boiling water and add to mixture.
3. Stir in oats and raisins.
4. Preheat the oven to 375 degrees F (190 degrees C). Line cookie sheets with parchment.
5. Roll the dough into balls or drop by tablespoonful, and place 2 inches apart on cookie sheets.
6. Bake for 8-10 minutes. Let cookies cool for 5 minutes before transferring to a wire rack.

44. Apple Crisp with Walnuts

Servings: 6

Total time: 50 minutes

Nutrition Facts

Serving Size 187 g

Amount Per Serving

Calories 332   Calories from Fat 131

              % Daily Value*

Total Fat 14.6g	**22%**
Saturated Fat 5.2g	**26%**
Trans Fat 0.0g	
Cholesterol 0mg	**0%**
Sodium 83mg	**3%**
Total Carbohydrates 48.2g	**16%**
Dietary Fiber 5.6g	**22%**
Sugars 30.8g	
Protein 5.8g	

Vitamin A 1%   •   Vitamin C 10%

Calcium 4%   •   Iron 5%

Nutrition Grade D+

* Based on a 2000 calorie diet

Ingredients

- 4 medium tart cooking apples, peeled, cored, and sliced (4 cups)
- ½ cup gluten-free all-purpose flour
- ¾ cup unrefined brown sugar
- ½ cup quick-cooking oats
- 1/5 teaspoon vanilla extract
- 1/3 cup softened low-fat butter
- ¾ teaspoon ground nutmeg
- ¾ teaspoon ground cinnamon
- 1/2 cup chopped walnuts

Directions

1. Preheat oven to 375 degrees F. Grease an 8-inch square pan with shortening.
2. Toss apples with half of the sugar and half of the cinnamon in a medium bowl; spread apples in pan. In a separate bowl, combine oats, flour, walnuts, and the remaining sugar and cinnamon. Using 2 forks or a pastry cutter, mash butter into the oats mixture until the mixture resembles coarse crumbs.

Spread oats mixture over apple mixture. Pat the topping gently until even.

3. Bake for 30 minutes or until apples are tender and topping is golden brown.

45. Low-Fat Berry Medley Parfait
Servings: 5
Total time: 55 minutes

Nutrition Facts

Serving Size 161 g

Amount Per Serving

Calories 268   Calories from Fat 98

	% Daily Value*
Total Fat 10.9g	**17%**
Saturated Fat 1.3g	**7%**
Trans Fat 0.0g	
Cholesterol 0mg	**0%**
Sodium 565mg	**24%**
Total Carbohydrates 17.8g	**6%**
Dietary Fiber 5.0g	**20%**
Sugars 6.3g	
Protein 14.3g	

Vitamin A 0%	•	Vitamin C 47%
Calcium 10%	•	Iron 6%

Nutrition Grade B+
* Based on a 2000 calorie diet

Ingredients
- 1 box(es) (3 oz) fat-free sugar-free wild strawberry gelatin
- 1 cup each sliced strawberries, blueberries and raspberries
- 2 cups prepared fat-free sugar-free vanilla pudding
- 1 cup chopped almonds (optional)

Directions
1. Prepare gelatin in a 2-cup glass measure as box directs and refrigerate for 30 minutes.
2. Divide berries evenly among five 10-oz glasses. Pour gelatin over the top of berries and gently stir to incorporate berries.
3. Refrigerate for 20 minutes until gelatin is set but not firm. Add the vanilla pudding on top of the gelatin-berries mixture.
4. Top each glass with almonds. Chill and serve.

About Robert M. Fleischer

Besides being a noted author, Robert M. Fleischer is a California-based health researcher, husband and a father of 2 children, both boys. He has dedicated his career to developing better standards of care and treatment for patients of common, chronic and misunderstood conditions which are often handled with pharmaceuticals to treat the symptoms rather than lifestyle changes which address the root cause.

In his spare time he enjoys archery, mountain biking and is a member of a local amateur theater group.

Exclusive Bonus Download: Nutrition Essentials

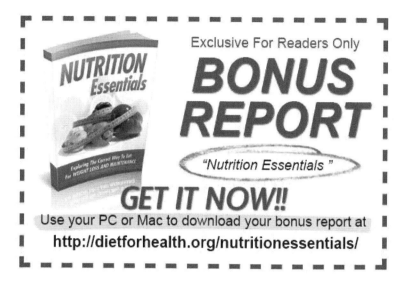

Download your bonus, please visit the download link above from your PC or MAC. To open PDF files, visit http://get.adobe.com/reader/ to download the reader if it's not already installed on your PC or Mac. To open ZIP files, you may need to download WinZip from http://www.winzip.com. This download is for PC or Mac ONLY and might not be downloadable to kindle.

Get All The Support And Guidance You Need To Be A Success At Understanding Nutrition!

Is the fact that you would like to get a grip on how to understand how to eat right for a healthy weight but just don't know how making your life difficult... maybe even miserable?

First, you are NOT alone! It may seem like it sometimes, but not knowing how to get started with nutrition for a healthy weight is far more common than you'd think.

Your lack of knowledge in this area may not be your fault, but that doesn't mean that you shouldn't -- or can't -- do anything to find out everything you need to know to finally be a success with understanding nutrition to have better health!

So today -- in the next FEW MINUTES, in fact -- we're going to help you GET ON TRACK, and learn how you can quickly and easily get your nutrition issues under control... for GOOD!

With this product, and it's great information on nutrition will walk you, step by step, through the exact process we developed to help people get all the info they need to be a success.

In This Book, You Will Learn:

- The Food Pyramid
- Correct Proteins For Weight Loss
- Correct Carbs For Weight Loss
- Correct Fats For Weight Loss
- What About Organic And Raw Foods
- And so much more!

Visit the URL above to download this guide and start living healthily NOW

One Last Thing...

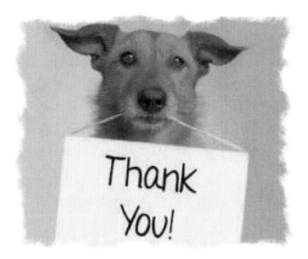

     Thank you so much for reading my book. I hope you really liked it. As you probably know, many people look at the reviews on Amazon before they decide to purchase a book. If you liked the book, could you please take a minute to leave a review with your feedback? 60 seconds is all I'm asking for, and it would mean the world to me.

Robert M. Fleischer

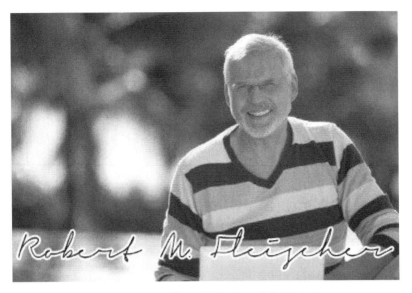

Copyright © 2012 Robert M. Fleischer

Images and Cover by NaturalWay Publishing

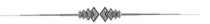

Atlanta, Georgia USA

Printed in Great Britain
by Amazon.co.uk, Ltd.,
Marston Gate.